THE
WORKOUT
JOURNAL
AND ROADMAP

TRACK • PROGRESS • ACHIEVE

CASTLE POINT BOOKS
NEW YORK

www.stmartins.com
www.castlepointbooks.com

The Castle Point Books trademark is owned by Castle Point Publishing, LLC.
Castle Point books are published and distributed by St. Martin's Press.

ISBN 978-1-250-19977-5 (trade paperback)

Design by Joanna Williams

Our books may be purchased in bulk for promotional, educational, or business use. Please contact your local bookseller or the Macmillan Corporate and Premium Sales Department at 1-800-221-7945, extension 5442, or by email at MacmillanSpecialMarkets@macmillan.com.

First Edition: December 2018

10 9 8 7 6 5 4

INSIDE

MAXIMIZE YOUR WORKOUTS **1**

SET S.M.A.R.T. GOALS **3**

WORKOUT AND FITNESS GOALS **4**

NUTRITION AND LIFESTYLE GOALS **5**

TIPS FOR TRACKING **7**

MARK YOUR START **9**

SEE PROGRESS **10**

WEEK 1..................................**12**
WEEK 2..................................**28**
WEEK 3..................................**44**
WEEK 4..................................**60**
WEEK 5..................................**76**
WEEK 6..................................**92**
WEEK 7................................**108**
WEEK 8................................**124**
WEEK 9................................**140**
WEEK 10..............................**156**
WEEK 11..............................**172**
WEEK 12..............................**188**
WEEK 13..............................**204**

"THE START
IS WHAT STOPS
MOST PEOPLE."

—DON SHULA

MAXIMIZE YOUR WORKOUTS

YOU'RE NOT MOST PEOPLE—you've committed to the start. But where will you finish? If you're ready to take your results farther than ever, it's time to get serious with your most powerful tool: *The Workout Journal and Roadmap!* The power lies in recording:

- **Your training goals**—whether it's more reps or sets with higher weight or going farther and faster with cardio, even flexibility and mobility goals

- **Where you are right now**—from body measurements to workout maxes and bests, so you can clearly see your progress and boost motivation to keep at it

- **Your performance for each workout**—celebrate successes (physical and mental) and troubleshoot anything holding you back

- **Extra support from nutrition, supplements, and sleep**— factors easy to overlook but also critical to reaching your fitness goals

The easy-to-use log pages that follow help you capture important workout measures—reps and sets, distance, heart rate, and more— in a strong, portable book. Plus, the simple yet powerful act of recording keeps you focused in each workout and motivated to stick to your overall fitness program. Get ready to see the results you've been chasing!

"SET YOUR GOALS
HIGH, AND DON'T STOP
TILL YOU GET THERE."

—BO JACKSON

SET S.M.A.R.T GOALS

EXPERTS AGREE THAT 90 DAYS is a smart, reasonable cycle in which you can set meaningful goals and expect great results. That's why this journal has been designed to cover 13 weeks—approximately 90 days. Your first step on that road to results: answering one all-important question. *Where do you want your workouts and nutrition plan to take you in the next 13 weeks?*

Before you get started, you need a destination in mind. As you name your targets, keep in mind that the best goals are S.M.A.R.T.:

- **Specific.** Don't set out to "lose weight;" aim to "lose inches off my waist."

- **Measureable.** Want to lift more weight? Aim to increase your bench press by a certain percentage or number of pounds.

- **Attainable.** While it's specific and measurable to set a goal of losing 10 percent body fat in 90 days, it's not attainable. Setting unreachable goals only sets you up for failure.

- **Realistic.** Even if a goal is technically attainable, it may not be realistic for you. If you haven't been training regularly, you're not going to be ready to compete in an Ironman triathlon in the next 90 days.

- **Timed.** You hold yourself accountable when you specify an end date—in this case, 13 weeks.

Ready to set your goals? Turn the page to start planning for results. You'll find space to record targets for fitness, nutrition, and even lifestyle (think about sleep, stress, and other factors that may affect your workouts).

WORKOUT AND FITNESS GOALS

GOAL	ACTION STEPS
GOAL	ACTION STEPS
GOAL	ACTION STEPS
GOAL	ACTION STEPS
GOAL	ACTION STEPS

FOR EACH GOAL, *outline key action steps it will take to get there. For example, if your fitness goal is to increase your weightlifting maxes by a certain percentage, how many workouts a week (including how many sets/reps) will it require? If your nutrition goal is to hit a daily protein target, what meals will you add to, and what foods will you zero in on?*

NUTRITION AND LIFESTYLE GOALS

GOAL	ACTION STEPS

GOAL	ACTION STEPS

GOAL	ACTION STEPS

GOAL	ACTION STEPS

GOAL	ACTION STEPS

"You cannot expect to build a
WELL-PROPORTIONED PHYSIQUE
without planning and following a
STRUCTURED ROUTINE."
—Simeon Panda

"OBSTACLES DON'T HAVE TO STOP YOU. IF YOU RUN INTO A WALL, DON'T TURN AROUND AND GIVE UP. FIGURE OUT HOW TO CLIMB IT, GO THROUGH IT, OR WORK AROUND IT."

—MICHAEL JORDAN

TIPS FOR TRACKING

NOW THAT YOU'VE SET YOUR GOALS, it's time to discover how using this journal can work hard to support them. For each of the 13 weeks, you'll find:

Weekly maps for your fitness and nutrition plans. Committing to specific action steps—workouts, meals, and more—on paper will help you head into the week with clear focus and motivation. (Meal planning can also save you time and money!) Spend time to make an outline at the beginning of each week, looking back at previous weeks to note what worked and what may need adjustment.

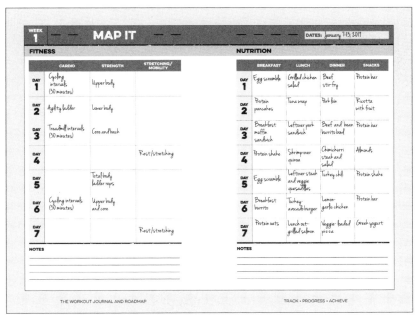

Daily tracker pages that give you a place to record how you followed through on your plan—the reality of how the day went. There's space for all kinds of workout measures, nutrition information for meals and snacks, supplements and water taken in, and sleep tracking. Each day, you can rate how well you stayed on target with your goals and make notes as to what worked and what didn't. You'll even get an expert tip or motivational quote to boost your results and resolve.

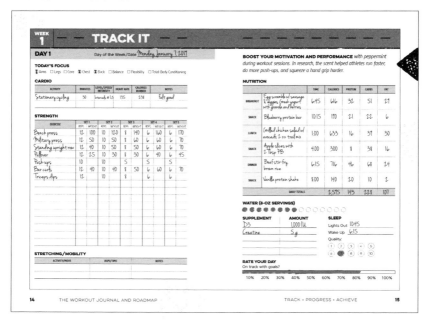

Weekly check-in charts (on pages 10–11) give you a great place to keep all your numbers together and see your successes add up. You'll be reminded to record your stats on day 7 of each training week. Track everything from chest, biceps, and waist measures to weight, body fat percentage, and resting heart rate—with space to add other factors important to you.

By keeping a detailed, complete journal, you will ensure that you are making progress toward your goals. If you're not getting where you want to go, your journal entries will have the answers to why you are not making progress. You can make adjustments and get right back on track!

MARK YOUR START

DATE: _____

Recording where you are now will help you see clear progress as you look back. Focus on the stats that are important to your goals.

BODY MEASUREMENTS

	CURRENT	GOAL	COMMENTS
NECK			
CHEST			
BICEPS			
WAIST			
HIPS			
THIGHS			
CALVES			
WEIGHT			
BODY FAT %			
RESTING HEART RATE			
BLOOD PRESSURE			
SLEEP QUALITY (1-10)			

WORKOUT BESTS

	CURRENT	GOAL	COMMENTS

NUTRITION NUMBERS

	CURRENT	GOAL	COMMENTS
CALORIES			
PROTEIN			
CARBS			
FAT			
WATER (8-OZ SERVINGS)			

WEEKLY CHECK-INS

	NECK	CHEST	BICEPS	WAIST	HIPS	THIGHS	CALVES	COMMENTS
WEEK 1 Date:___								
WEEK 2 Date:___								
WEEK 3 Date:___								
WEEK 4 Date:___								
WEEK 5 Date:___								
WEEK 6 Date:___								
WEEK 7 Date:___								
WEEK 8 Date:___								
WEEK 9 Date:___								
WEEK 10 Date:___								
WEEK 11 Date:___								
WEEK 12 Date:___								
WEEK 13 Date:___								

WEEKLY CHECK-INS

	WEIGHT	BODY FAT %	RESTING HEART RATE	BLOOD PRESSURE	SLEEP QUALITY (1-10)			COMMENTS
WEEK 1 Date:___								
WEEK 2 Date:___								
WEEK 3 Date:___								
WEEK 4 Date:___								
WEEK 5 Date:___								
WEEK 6 Date:___								
WEEK 7 Date:___								
WEEK 8 Date:___								
WEEK 9 Date:___								
WEEK 10 Date:___								
WEEK 11 Date:___								
WEEK 12 Date:___								
WEEK 13 Date:___								

MAP IT

FITNESS

	CARDIO	STRENGTH	STRETCHING/ MOBILITY
DAY 1			
DAY 2			
DAY 3			
DAY 4			
DAY 5			
DAY 6			
DAY 7			

NOTES

_____

_____

_____

_____

NUTRITION

	BREAKFAST	LUNCH	DINNER	SNACKS
DAY 1				
DAY 2				
DAY 3				
DAY 4				
DAY 5				
DAY 6				
DAY 7				

NOTES

DAY 1

Day of the Week/Date _____

TODAY'S FOCUS

☐ Arms ☐ Legs ☐ Core ☐ Chest ☐ Back ☐ Balance ☐ Flexibility ☐ Total-Body Conditioning

CARDIO

ACTIVITY	MINUTES	LEVEL/SPEED/INTENSITY	HEART RATE	CALORIES BURNED	NOTES

STRENGTH

EXERCISE	SET 1		SET 2		SET 3		SET 4		SET 5	
	REPS	WEIGHT	REPS	WEIGHT	REPS	WEIGHT	REPS	WEIGHT	REPS	WEIGHT

STRETCHING/MOBILITY

ACTIVITY/MOVE	REPS/TIME	NOTES

BOOST YOUR MOTIVATION AND PERFORMANCE *with peppermint during workout sessions. In research, the scent helped athletes run faster, do more push-ups, and squeeze a hand grip harder.*

NUTRITION

		TIME	CALORIES	PROTEIN	CARBS	FAT
BREAKFAST						
SNACK						
LUNCH						
SNACK						
DINNER						
SNACK						
DAILY TOTALS						

WATER (8-OZ SERVINGS)

○ ○ ○ ○ ○ ○ ○ ○ ○ ○ ○ ○ ○ ○ ○

SUPPLEMENT   **AMOUNT**

_____ | _____

_____ | _____

_____ | _____

_____ | _____

_____ | _____

SLEEP

Lights Out _____

Wake Up _____

Quality:

① ② ③ ④ ⑤

⑥ ⑦ ⑧ ⑨ ⑩

RATE YOUR DAY
On track with goals?

| 10% | 20% | 30% | 40% | 50% | 60% | 70% | 80% | 90% | 100% |

DAY 2   Day of the Week/Date _____

TODAY'S FOCUS
☐ Arms   ☐ Legs   ☐ Core   ☐ Chest   ☐ Back   ☐ Balance   ☐ Flexibility   ☐ Total-Body Conditioning

CARDIO

ACTIVITY	MINUTES	LEVEL/SPEED/ INTENSITY	HEART RATE	CALORIES BURNED	NOTES

STRENGTH

EXERCISE	SET 1		SET 2		SET 3		SET 4		SET 5	
	REPS	WEIGHT	REPS	WEIGHT	REPS	WEIGHT	REPS	WEIGHT	REPS	WEIGHT

STRETCHING/MOBILITY

ACTIVITY/MOVE	REPS/TIME	NOTES

COUNT BACKWARD FOR GAINS. *It's a sneaky little trick for tracking reps that makes it easier to stay mentally and physically strong and push out those last tough ones.*

NUTRITION

		TIME	CALORIES	PROTEIN	CARBS	FAT
BREAKFAST						
SNACK						
LUNCH						
SNACK						
DINNER						
SNACK						
DAILY TOTALS						

WATER (8-OZ SERVINGS)

○ ○ ○ ○ ○ ○ ○ ○ ○ ○ ○ ○ ○ ○ ○

SUPPLEMENT	AMOUNT
_____	_____
_____	_____
_____	_____
_____	_____
_____	_____

SLEEP

Lights Out _____

Wake Up _____

Quality:

① ② ③ ④ ⑤
⑥ ⑦ ⑧ ⑨ ⑩

RATE YOUR DAY
On track with goals?

| 10% | 20% | 30% | 40% | 50% | 60% | 70% | 80% | 90% | 100% |

DAY 3

Day of the Week/Date _____

TODAY'S FOCUS

☐ Arms ☐ Legs ☐ Core ☐ Chest ☐ Back ☐ Balance ☐ Flexibility ☐ Total-Body Conditioning

CARDIO

ACTIVITY	MINUTES	LEVEL/SPEED/INTENSITY	HEART RATE	CALORIES BURNED	NOTES

STRENGTH

EXERCISE	SET 1		SET 2		SET 3		SET 4		SET 5	
	REPS	WEIGHT	REPS	WEIGHT	REPS	WEIGHT	REPS	WEIGHT	REPS	WEIGHT

STRETCHING/MOBILITY

ACTIVITY/MOVE	REPS/TIME	NOTES

ALWAYS FINISH STRONG.
"There are better starters than me but I'm a strong finisher." —*Usain Bolt*

NUTRITION

		TIME	CALORIES	PROTEIN	CARBS	FAT
BREAKFAST						
SNACK						
LUNCH						
SNACK						
DINNER						
SNACK						
DAILY TOTALS						

WATER (8-OZ SERVINGS)
○ ○ ○ ○ ○ ○ ○ ○ ○ ○ ○ ○ ○ ○ ○ ○

SUPPLEMENT   **AMOUNT**

_____ | _____
_____ | _____
_____ | _____
_____ | _____
_____ | _____

SLEEP

Lights Out _____

Wake Up _____

Quality:

(1) (2) (3) (4) (5)

(6) (7) (8) (9) (10)

RATE YOUR DAY
On track with goals?

| 10% | 20% | 30% | 40% | 50% | 60% | 70% | 80% | 90% | 100% |

DAY 4

Day of the Week/Date _____

TODAY'S FOCUS

☐ Arms ☐ Legs ☐ Core ☐ Chest ☐ Back ☐ Balance ☐ Flexibility ☐ Total-Body Conditioning

CARDIO

ACTIVITY	MINUTES	LEVEL/SPEED/ INTENSITY	HEART RATE	CALORIES BURNED	NOTES

STRENGTH

EXERCISE	SET 1		SET 2		SET 3		SET 4		SET 5	
	REPS	WEIGHT	REPS	WEIGHT	REPS	WEIGHT	REPS	WEIGHT	REPS	WEIGHT

STRETCHING/MOBILITY

ACTIVITY/MOVE	REPS/TIME	NOTES

TREAT TIRED MUSCLES *to a chug of chocolate milk. Research shows it's a stellar recovery drink after a tough workout, with its high carb and protein content and just a touch of sugar and sodium.*

NUTRITION

		TIME	CALORIES	PROTEIN	CARBS	FAT
BREAKFAST						
SNACK						
LUNCH						
SNACK						
DINNER						
SNACK						
DAILY TOTALS						

WATER (8-OZ SERVINGS)

○ ○ ○ ○ ○ ○ ○ ○ ○ ○ ○ ○ ○ ○ ○

SUPPLEMENT	AMOUNT
_____	_____
_____	_____
_____	_____
_____	_____
_____	_____

SLEEP

Lights Out _____

Wake Up _____

Quality:

① ② ③ ④ ⑤
⑥ ⑦ ⑧ ⑨ ⑩

RATE YOUR DAY
On track with goals?

| 10% | 20% | 30% | 40% | 50% | 60% | 70% | 80% | 90% | 100% |

TRACK IT

DAY 5

Day of the Week/Date _____

TODAY'S FOCUS

☐ Arms ☐ Legs ☐ Core ☐ Chest ☐ Back ☐ Balance ☐ Flexibility ☐ Total-Body Conditioning

CARDIO

ACTIVITY	MINUTES	LEVEL/SPEED/INTENSITY	HEART RATE	CALORIES BURNED	NOTES

STRENGTH

EXERCISE	SET 1		SET 2		SET 3		SET 4		SET 5	
	REPS	WEIGHT	REPS	WEIGHT	REPS	WEIGHT	REPS	WEIGHT	REPS	WEIGHT

STRETCHING/MOBILITY

ACTIVITY/MOVE	REPS/TIME	NOTES

LIFT IN ORDER. *Go to dumbbells first, then barbells, and finally machines. Your smaller stabilizer muscles will have more energy for dumbbells at the start. Machines call on larger muscle groups that have more staying power.*

NUTRITION

		TIME	CALORIES	PROTEIN	CARBS	FAT
BREAKFAST						
SNACK						
LUNCH						
SNACK						
DINNER						
SNACK						
DAILY TOTALS						

WATER (8-OZ SERVINGS)

○ ○ ○ ○ ○ ○ ○ ○ ○ ○ ○ ○ ○ ○ ○

SUPPLEMENT	AMOUNT
_____	_____
_____	_____
_____	_____
_____	_____
_____	_____

SLEEP

Lights Out _____

Wake Up _____

Quality:

① ② ③ ④ ⑤
⑥ ⑦ ⑧ ⑨ ⑩

RATE YOUR DAY
On track with goals?

10% 20% 30% 40% 50% 60% 70% 80% 90% 100%

TRACK IT

DAY 6　　　　Day of the Week/Date _____

TODAY'S FOCUS

☐ Arms　☐ Legs　☐ Core　☐ Chest　☐ Back　☐ Balance　☐ Flexibility　☐ Total-Body Conditioning

CARDIO

ACTIVITY	MINUTES	LEVEL/SPEED/INTENSITY	HEART RATE	CALORIES BURNED	NOTES

STRENGTH

EXERCISE	SET 1		SET 2		SET 3		SET 4		SET 5	
	REPS	WEIGHT	REPS	WEIGHT	REPS	WEIGHT	REPS	WEIGHT	REPS	WEIGHT

STRETCHING/MOBILITY

ACTIVITY/MOVE	REPS/TIME	NOTES

NO EXCUSES!

"Ninety-nine percent of failures come from people who have the habit of making excuses." —*George W. Carver*

NUTRITION

	TIME	CALORIES	PROTEIN	CARBS	FAT
BREAKFAST					
SNACK					
LUNCH					
SNACK					
DINNER					
SNACK					
DAILY TOTALS					

WATER (8-OZ SERVINGS)

○ ○ ○ ○ ○ ○ ○ ○ ○ ○ ○ ○ ○ ○ ○

SUPPLEMENT	AMOUNT

SLEEP

Lights Out _____

Wake Up _____

Quality:

① ② ③ ④ ⑤
⑥ ⑦ ⑧ ⑨ ⑩

RATE YOUR DAY

On track with goals?

| 10% | 20% | 30% | 40% | 50% | 60% | 70% | 80% | 90% | 100% |

DAY 7

Day of the Week/Date _____

TODAY'S FOCUS

☐ Arms ☐ Legs ☐ Core ☐ Chest ☐ Back ☐ Balance ☐ Flexibility ☐ Total-Body Conditioning

CARDIO

ACTIVITY	MINUTES	LEVEL/SPEED/INTENSITY	HEART RATE	CALORIES BURNED	NOTES

STRENGTH

EXERCISE	SET 1		SET 2		SET 3		SET 4		SET 5	
	REPS	WEIGHT	REPS	WEIGHT	REPS	WEIGHT	REPS	WEIGHT	REPS	WEIGHT

STRETCHING/MOBILITY

ACTIVITY/MOVE	REPS/TIME	NOTES

GOAL CHECK! *Now that you've reached the end of your first journaling week, don't forget to log the start of your results in "See Progress" on pages 10 and 11.*

NUTRITION

		TIME	CALORIES	PROTEIN	CARBS	FAT
BREAKFAST						
SNACK						
LUNCH						
SNACK						
DINNER						
SNACK						
	DAILY TOTALS					

WATER (8-OZ SERVINGS)

○ ○ ○ ○ ○ ○ ○ ○ ○ ○ ○ ○ ○ ○ ○ ○

SUPPLEMENT	**AMOUNT**
_____	_____
_____	_____
_____	_____
_____	_____
_____	_____

SLEEP

Lights Out _____

Wake Up _____

Quality:

① ② ③ ④ ⑤
⑥ ⑦ ⑧ ⑨ ⑩

RATE YOUR DAY
On track with goals?

| 10% | 20% | 30% | 40% | 50% | 60% | 70% | 80% | 90% | 100% |

FITNESS

	CARDIO	STRENGTH	STRETCHING/ MOBILITY
DAY 1			
DAY 2			
DAY 3			
DAY 4			
DAY 5			
DAY 6			
DAY 7			

NOTES

_____
_____
_____
_____

NUTRITION

	BREAKFAST	LUNCH	DINNER	SNACKS
DAY 1				
DAY 2				
DAY 3				
DAY 4				
DAY 5				
DAY 6				
DAY 7				

NOTES

TRACK IT

DAY 1

Day of the Week/Date _____

TODAY'S FOCUS

☐ Arms ☐ Legs ☐ Core ☐ Chest ☐ Back ☐ Balance ☐ Flexibility ☐ Total-Body Conditioning

CARDIO

ACTIVITY	MINUTES	LEVEL/SPEED/INTENSITY	HEART RATE	CALORIES BURNED	NOTES

STRENGTH

EXERCISE	SET 1		SET 2		SET 3		SET 4		SET 5	
	REPS	WEIGHT	REPS	WEIGHT	REPS	WEIGHT	REPS	WEIGHT	REPS	WEIGHT

STRETCHING/MOBILITY

ACTIVITY/MOVE	REPS/TIME	NOTES

GET A KICK FROM COFFEE. *A 16-ounce cup of coffee about an hour before a workout can help boost your endurance and make exercise feel easier. Chase it with 6 to 8 ounces of water for best results.*

NUTRITION

		TIME	CALORIES	PROTEIN	CARBS	FAT
BREAKFAST						
SNACK						
LUNCH						
SNACK						
DINNER						
SNACK						
DAILY TOTALS						

WATER (8-OZ SERVINGS)

○ ○ ○ ○ ○ ○ ○ ○ ○ ○ ○ ○ ○ ○ ○ ○

SUPPLEMENT	AMOUNT
_____	_____
_____	_____
_____	_____
_____	_____
_____	_____

SLEEP

Lights Out _____

Wake Up _____

Quality:

① ② ③ ④ ⑤
⑥ ⑦ ⑧ ⑨ ⑩

RATE YOUR DAY
On track with goals?

| 10% | 20% | 30% | 40% | 50% | 60% | 70% | 80% | 90% | 100% |

TRACK IT

DAY 2

Day of the Week/Date _____

TODAY'S FOCUS

☐ Arms ☐ Legs ☐ Core ☐ Chest ☐ Back ☐ Balance ☐ Flexibility ☐ Total-Body Conditioning

CARDIO

ACTIVITY	MINUTES	LEVEL/SPEED/INTENSITY	HEART RATE	CALORIES BURNED	NOTES

STRENGTH

EXERCISE	SET 1		SET 2		SET 3		SET 4		SET 5	
	REPS	WEIGHT	REPS	WEIGHT	REPS	WEIGHT	REPS	WEIGHT	REPS	WEIGHT

STRETCHING/MOBILITY

ACTIVITY/MOVE	REPS/TIME	NOTES

WATCH THE WEIGHT BELT. *It's not going to help (and could block gains) when performing crunches or simple moves such as biceps curls. Save it for maximal lifts in exercises such as squats, deadlifts, and overhead presses.*

NUTRITION

		TIME	CALORIES	PROTEIN	CARBS	FAT
BREAKFAST						
SNACK						
LUNCH						
SNACK						
DINNER						
SNACK						
DAILY TOTALS						

WATER (8-OZ SERVINGS)

○ ○ ○ ○ ○ ○ ○ ○ ○ ○ ○ ○ ○ ○ ○

SUPPLEMENT | AMOUNT

_____ | _____

_____ | _____

_____ | _____

_____ | _____

_____ | _____

SLEEP

Lights Out _____

Wake Up _____

Quality:

① ② ③ ④ ⑤

⑥ ⑦ ⑧ ⑨ ⑩

RATE YOUR DAY

On track with goals?

| 10% | 20% | 30% | 40% | 50% | 60% | 70% | 80% | 90% | 100% |

DAY 3

Day of the Week/Date _____

TODAY'S FOCUS

☐ Arms ☐ Legs ☐ Core ☐ Chest ☐ Back ☐ Balance ☐ Flexibility ☐ Total-Body Conditioning

CARDIO

ACTIVITY	MINUTES	LEVEL/SPEED/INTENSITY	HEART RATE	CALORIES BURNED	NOTES

STRENGTH

EXERCISE	SET 1		SET 2		SET 3		SET 4		SET 5	
	REPS	WEIGHT	REPS	WEIGHT	REPS	WEIGHT	REPS	WEIGHT	REPS	WEIGHT

STRETCHING/MOBILITY

ACTIVITY/MOVE	REPS/TIME	NOTES

KEEP IT UP.

"Be very strong...be very methodical in your life if you want to be a champion." —Alberto Juantorena

NUTRITION

		TIME	CALORIES	PROTEIN	CARBS	FAT
BREAKFAST						
SNACK						
LUNCH						
SNACK						
DINNER						
SNACK						
	DAILY TOTALS					

WATER (8-OZ SERVINGS)

○ ○ ○ ○ ○ ○ ○ ○ ○ ○ ○ ○ ○ ○ ○

SUPPLEMENT	AMOUNT
_____	_____
_____	_____
_____	_____
_____	_____
_____	_____

SLEEP

Lights Out _____

Wake Up _____

Quality:

① ② ③ ④ ⑤
⑥ ⑦ ⑧ ⑨ ⑩

RATE YOUR DAY

On track with goals?

| 10% | 20% | 30% | 40% | 50% | 60% | 70% | 80% | 90% | 100% |

DAY 4

Day of the Week/Date _____

TODAY'S FOCUS

☐ Arms ☐ Legs ☐ Core ☐ Chest ☐ Back ☐ Balance ☐ Flexibility ☐ Total-Body Conditioning

CARDIO

ACTIVITY	MINUTES	LEVEL/SPEED/INTENSITY	HEART RATE	CALORIES BURNED	NOTES

STRENGTH

EXERCISE	SET 1		SET 2		SET 3		SET 4		SET 5	
	REPS	WEIGHT	REPS	WEIGHT	REPS	WEIGHT	REPS	WEIGHT	REPS	WEIGHT

STRETCHING/MOBILITY

ACTIVITY/MOVE	REPS/TIME	NOTES

USE THE FORMULA FOR MORE MUSCLE. *Multiply the weight you lift by your total reps completed for an exercise. Try to increase that number every workout by lifting more weight, increasing your reps, or completing more sets.*

NUTRITION

		TIME	CALORIES	PROTEIN	CARBS	FAT
BREAKFAST						
SNACK						
LUNCH						
SNACK						
DINNER						
SNACK						
DAILY TOTALS						

WATER (8-OZ SERVINGS)

○ ○ ○ ○ ○ ○ ○ ○ ○ ○ ○ ○ ○ ○ ○ ○

SUPPLEMENT   **AMOUNT**

_____ _____

_____ _____

_____ _____

_____ _____

_____ _____

SLEEP

Lights Out _____

Wake Up _____

Quality:

① ② ③ ④ ⑤
⑥ ⑦ ⑧ ⑨ ⑩

RATE YOUR DAY
On track with goals?

| 10% | 20% | 30% | 40% | 50% | 60% | 70% | 80% | 90% | 100% |

DAY 5

Day of the Week/Date _____

TODAY'S FOCUS

☐ Arms ☐ Legs ☐ Core ☐ Chest ☐ Back ☐ Balance ☐ Flexibility ☐ Total-Body Conditioning

CARDIO

ACTIVITY	MINUTES	LEVEL/SPEED/INTENSITY	HEART RATE	CALORIES BURNED	NOTES

STRENGTH

EXERCISE	SET 1		SET 2		SET 3		SET 4		SET 5	
	REPS	WEIGHT	REPS	WEIGHT	REPS	WEIGHT	REPS	WEIGHT	REPS	WEIGHT

STRETCHING/MOBILITY

ACTIVITY/MOVE	REPS/TIME	NOTES

NEED ANOTHER REASON TO LIFT? *It gives you a mental lift. Researchers at the University of Limerick, Ireland, found that strength training can significantly reduce depression symptoms among adults.*

NUTRITION

	TIME	CALORIES	PROTEIN	CARBS	FAT
BREAKFAST					
SNACK					
LUNCH					
SNACK					
DINNER					
SNACK					
DAILY TOTALS					

WATER (8-OZ SERVINGS)

○ ○ ○ ○ ○ ○ ○ ○ ○ ○ ○ ○ ○ ○ ○ ○

SUPPLEMENT   **AMOUNT**

_____ | _____
_____ | _____
_____ | _____
_____ | _____
_____ | _____

SLEEP

Lights Out _____

Wake Up _____

Quality:

① ② ③ ④ ⑤
⑥ ⑦ ⑧ ⑨ ⑩

RATE YOUR DAY
On track with goals?

| 10% | 20% | 30% | 40% | 50% | 60% | 70% | 80% | 90% | 100% |

TRACK IT

DAY 6

Day of the Week/Date _____

TODAY'S FOCUS

☐ Arms ☐ Legs ☐ Core ☐ Chest ☐ Back ☐ Balance ☐ Flexibility ☐ Total-Body Conditioning

CARDIO

ACTIVITY	MINUTES	LEVEL/SPEED/INTENSITY	HEART RATE	CALORIES BURNED	NOTES

STRENGTH

EXERCISE	SET 1		SET 2		SET 3		SET 4		SET 5	
	REPS	WEIGHT	REPS	WEIGHT	REPS	WEIGHT	REPS	WEIGHT	REPS	WEIGHT

STRETCHING/MOBILITY

ACTIVITY/MOVE	REPS/TIME	NOTES

AIM HIGH.

"You have to expect things of yourself before you can do them."
—Michael Jordan

NUTRITION

		TIME	CALORIES	PROTEIN	CARBS	FAT
BREAKFAST						
SNACK						
LUNCH						
SNACK						
DINNER						
SNACK						
DAILY TOTALS						

WATER (8-OZ SERVINGS)

○ ○ ○ ○ ○ ○ ○ ○ ○ ○ ○ ○ ○ ○ ○

SUPPLEMENT	AMOUNT
_____	_____
_____	_____
_____	_____
_____	_____
_____	_____

SLEEP

Lights Out _____

Wake Up _____

Quality:

① ② ③ ④ ⑤
⑥ ⑦ ⑧ ⑨ ⑩

RATE YOUR DAY

On track with goals?

| 10% | 20% | 30% | 40% | 50% | 60% | 70% | 80% | 90% | 100% |

TRACK IT

DAY 7

Day of the Week/Date _____

TODAY'S FOCUS

☐ Arms ☐ Legs ☐ Core ☐ Chest ☐ Back ☐ Balance ☐ Flexibility ☐ Total-Body Conditioning

CARDIO

ACTIVITY	MINUTES	LEVEL/SPEED/INTENSITY	HEART RATE	CALORIES BURNED	NOTES

STRENGTH

EXERCISE	SET 1		SET 2		SET 3		SET 4		SET 5	
	REPS	WEIGHT	REPS	WEIGHT	REPS	WEIGHT	REPS	WEIGHT	REPS	WEIGHT

STRETCHING/MOBILITY

ACTIVITY/MOVE	REPS/TIME	NOTES

WEEK 2 IS IN THE BOOKS! *Take a few minutes to log your numbers in "See Progress" on pages 10 and 11.*

NUTRITION

		TIME	CALORIES	PROTEIN	CARBS	FAT
BREAKFAST						
SNACK						
LUNCH						
SNACK						
DINNER						
SNACK						
DAILY TOTALS						

WATER (8-OZ SERVINGS)

○ ○ ○ ○ ○ ○ ○ ○ ○ ○ ○ ○ ○ ○ ○

SUPPLEMENT	AMOUNT
_____	_____
_____	_____
_____	_____
_____	_____
_____	_____

SLEEP

Lights Out _____

Wake Up _____

Quality:

① ② ③ ④ ⑤
⑥ ⑦ ⑧ ⑨ ⑩

RATE YOUR DAY
On track with goals?

| 10% | 20% | 30% | 40% | 50% | 60% | 70% | 80% | 90% | 100% |

MAP IT

FITNESS

	CARDIO	STRENGTH	STRETCHING/ MOBILITY
DAY 1			
DAY 2			
DAY 3			
DAY 4			
DAY 5			
DAY 6			
DAY 7			

NOTES

_____
_____
_____
_____

NUTRITION

	BREAKFAST	LUNCH	DINNER	SNACKS
DAY 1				
DAY 2				
DAY 3				
DAY 4				
DAY 5				
DAY 6				
DAY 7				

NOTES

DAY 1

Day of the Week/Date _____

TODAY'S FOCUS

☐ Arms   ☐ Legs   ☐ Core   ☐ Chest   ☐ Back   ☐ Balance   ☐ Flexibility   ☐ Total-Body Conditioning

CARDIO

ACTIVITY	MINUTES	LEVEL/SPEED/INTENSITY	HEART RATE	CALORIES BURNED	NOTES

STRENGTH

EXERCISE	SET 1		SET 2		SET 3		SET 4		SET 5	
	REPS	WEIGHT	REPS	WEIGHT	REPS	WEIGHT	REPS	WEIGHT	REPS	WEIGHT

STRETCHING/MOBILITY

ACTIVITY/MOVE	REPS/TIME	NOTES

STRENGTHEN YOUR SQUAT. *The adjustment that makes the difference: Simply standing in front of the bench when you squat. Pretend you're about to sit down. It'll help you go lower while keeping impressive form.*

NUTRITION

	TIME	CALORIES	PROTEIN	CARBS	FAT
BREAKFAST					
SNACK					
LUNCH					
SNACK					
DINNER					
SNACK					
DAILY TOTALS					

WATER (8-OZ SERVINGS)

○ ○ ○ ○ ○ ○ ○ ○ ○ ○ ○ ○ ○ ○ ○ ○

SUPPLEMENT   **AMOUNT**

_____ | _____

_____ | _____

_____ | _____

_____ | _____

_____ | _____

SLEEP

Lights Out _____

Wake Up _____

Quality:

① ② ③ ④ ⑤
⑥ ⑦ ⑧ ⑨ ⑩

RATE YOUR DAY
On track with goals?

| 10% | 20% | 30% | 40% | 50% | 60% | 70% | 80% | 90% | 100% |

DAY 2

Day of the Week/Date _____

TODAY'S FOCUS

☐ Arms ☐ Legs ☐ Core ☐ Chest ☐ Back ☐ Balance ☐ Flexibility ☐ Total-Body Conditioning

CARDIO

ACTIVITY	MINUTES	LEVEL/SPEED/INTENSITY	HEART RATE	CALORIES BURNED	NOTES

STRENGTH

EXERCISE	SET 1		SET 2		SET 3		SET 4		SET 5	
	REPS	WEIGHT	REPS	WEIGHT	REPS	WEIGHT	REPS	WEIGHT	REPS	WEIGHT

STRETCHING/MOBILITY

ACTIVITY/MOVE	REPS/TIME	NOTES

YOU NEED GYM BUDDIES! *Lift a small wave, nod your head, ask for a spot, or simply grunt a greeting, if that's all you can muster. Familiar faces can keep you coming back on days when motivation is low.*

NUTRITION

		TIME	CALORIES	PROTEIN	CARBS	FAT
BREAKFAST						
SNACK						
LUNCH						
SNACK						
DINNER						
SNACK						
DAILY TOTALS						

WATER (8-OZ SERVINGS)

○ ○ ○ ○ ○ ○ ○ ○ ○ ○ ○ ○ ○ ○ ○

SUPPLEMENT   **AMOUNT**

_____ | _____
_____ | _____
_____ | _____
_____ | _____
_____ | _____

SLEEP

Lights Out _____
Wake Up _____
Quality:

① ② ③ ④ ⑤
⑥ ⑦ ⑧ ⑨ ⑩

RATE YOUR DAY
On track with goals?

| 10% | 20% | 30% | 40% | 50% | 60% | 70% | 80% | 90% | 100% |

TRACK IT

DAY 3

Day of the Week/Date _____

TODAY'S FOCUS

☐ Arms   ☐ Legs   ☐ Core   ☐ Chest   ☐ Back   ☐ Balance   ☐ Flexibility   ☐ Total-Body Conditioning

CARDIO

ACTIVITY	MINUTES	LEVEL/SPEED/INTENSITY	HEART RATE	CALORIES BURNED	NOTES

STRENGTH

EXERCISE	SET 1		SET 2		SET 3		SET 4		SET 5	
	REPS	WEIGHT	REPS	WEIGHT	REPS	WEIGHT	REPS	WEIGHT	REPS	WEIGHT

STRETCHING/MOBILITY

ACTIVITY/MOVE	REPS/TIME	NOTES

GO BIG AND BOLD.

"To uncover your true potential you must first find your own limits and then you have to have the courage to blow past them." —*Picabo Street*

NUTRITION

		TIME	CALORIES	PROTEIN	CARBS	FAT
BREAKFAST						
SNACK						
LUNCH						
SNACK						
DINNER						
SNACK						
DAILY TOTALS						

WATER (8-OZ SERVINGS)

○ ○ ○ ○ ○ ○ ○ ○ ○ ○ ○ ○ ○ ○ ○

SUPPLEMENT	AMOUNT
_____	_____
_____	_____
_____	_____
_____	_____
_____	_____

SLEEP

Lights Out _____

Wake Up _____

Quality:

① ② ③ ④ ⑤
⑥ ⑦ ⑧ ⑨ ⑩

RATE YOUR DAY

On track with goals?

| 10% | 20% | 30% | 40% | 50% | 60% | 70% | 80% | 90% | 100% |

TRACK IT

DAY 4   Day of the Week/Date _____

TODAY'S FOCUS

☐ Arms ☐ Legs ☐ Core ☐ Chest ☐ Back ☐ Balance ☐ Flexibility ☐ Total-Body Conditioning

CARDIO

ACTIVITY	MINUTES	LEVEL/SPEED/INTENSITY	HEART RATE	CALORIES BURNED	NOTES

STRENGTH

EXERCISE	SET 1		SET 2		SET 3		SET 4		SET 5	
	REPS	WEIGHT	REPS	WEIGHT	REPS	WEIGHT	REPS	WEIGHT	REPS	WEIGHT

STRETCHING/MOBILITY

ACTIVITY/MOVE	REPS/TIME	NOTES

KNOW YOUR PROTEIN NEEDS. *Researchers who looked at 49 studies concluded that consuming up to 0.73 grams of protein per pound of body weight per day is ideal for building muscle.*

NUTRITION

		TIME	CALORIES	PROTEIN	CARBS	FAT
BREAKFAST						
SNACK						
LUNCH						
SNACK						
DINNER						
SNACK						
DAILY TOTALS						

WATER (8-OZ SERVINGS)
○ ○ ○ ○ ○ ○ ○ ○ ○ ○ ○ ○ ○ ○ ○ ○

SUPPLEMENT	AMOUNT
_____	_____
_____	_____
_____	_____
_____	_____
_____	_____

SLEEP

Lights Out _____

Wake Up _____

Quality:

(1) (2) (3) (4) (5)

(6) (7) (8) (9) (10)

RATE YOUR DAY
On track with goals?

| 10% | 20% | 30% | 40% | 50% | 60% | 70% | 80% | 90% | 100% |

TRACK IT

DAY 5

Day of the Week/Date _____

TODAY'S FOCUS

☐ Arms ☐ Legs ☐ Core ☐ Chest ☐ Back ☐ Balance ☐ Flexibility ☐ Total-Body Conditioning

CARDIO

ACTIVITY	MINUTES	LEVEL/SPEED/INTENSITY	HEART RATE	CALORIES BURNED	NOTES

STRENGTH

EXERCISE	SET 1		SET 2		SET 3		SET 4		SET 5	
	REPS	WEIGHT	REPS	WEIGHT	REPS	WEIGHT	REPS	WEIGHT	REPS	WEIGHT

STRETCHING/MOBILITY

ACTIVITY/MOVE	REPS/TIME	NOTES

SOOTHE SORE MUSCLES. *Try adding yellow mustard—anywhere from a few tablespoons to a whole 8-ounce bottle—to a hot bath. The bathwater may look strange, but your sore muscles will feel ready to hit the gym again sooner.*

NUTRITION

		TIME	CALORIES	PROTEIN	CARBS	FAT
BREAKFAST						
SNACK						
LUNCH						
SNACK						
DINNER						
SNACK						
DAILY TOTALS						

WATER (8-OZ SERVINGS)

○ ○ ○ ○ ○ ○ ○ ○ ○ ○ ○ ○ ○ ○ ○

SUPPLEMENT	AMOUNT
_____	_____
_____	_____
_____	_____
_____	_____
_____	_____

SLEEP

Lights Out _____

Wake Up _____

Quality:

① ② ③ ④ ⑤
⑥ ⑦ ⑧ ⑨ ⑩

RATE YOUR DAY
On track with goals?

| 10% | 20% | 30% | 40% | 50% | 60% | 70% | 80% | 90% | 100% |

TRACK IT

DAY 6

Day of the Week/Date _____

TODAY'S FOCUS

☐ Arms ☐ Legs ☐ Core ☐ Chest ☐ Back ☐ Balance ☐ Flexibility ☐ Total-Body Conditioning

CARDIO

ACTIVITY	MINUTES	LEVEL/SPEED/INTENSITY	HEART RATE	CALORIES BURNED	NOTES

STRENGTH

EXERCISE	SET 1		SET 2		SET 3		SET 4		SET 5	
	REPS	WEIGHT	REPS	WEIGHT	REPS	WEIGHT	REPS	WEIGHT	REPS	WEIGHT

STRETCHING/MOBILITY

ACTIVITY/MOVE	REPS/TIME	NOTES

WHEN YOU STRUGGLE, REMEMBER:
"The only bad workout is the one that didn't happen." —*Anonymous*

NUTRITION

		TIME	CALORIES	PROTEIN	CARBS	FAT
BREAKFAST						
SNACK						
LUNCH						
SNACK						
DINNER						
SNACK						
	DAILY TOTALS					

WATER (8-OZ SERVINGS)

○ ○ ○ ○ ○ ○ ○ ○ ○ ○ ○ ○ ○ ○ ○ ○

SUPPLEMENT   **AMOUNT**

_____ | _____
_____ | _____
_____ | _____
_____ | _____
_____ | _____

SLEEP

Lights Out _____
Wake Up _____
Quality:

① ② ③ ④ ⑤
⑥ ⑦ ⑧ ⑨ ⑩

RATE YOUR DAY
On track with goals?

10%   20%   30%   40%   50%   60%   70%   80%   90%   100%

TRACK IT

DAY 7

Day of the Week/Date _____

TODAY'S FOCUS

☐ Arms ☐ Legs ☐ Core ☐ Chest ☐ Back ☐ Balance ☐ Flexibility ☐ Total-Body Conditioning

CARDIO

ACTIVITY	MINUTES	LEVEL/SPEED/INTENSITY	HEART RATE	CALORIES BURNED	NOTES

STRENGTH

EXERCISE	SET 1		SET 2		SET 3		SET 4		SET 5	
	REPS	WEIGHT	REPS	WEIGHT	REPS	WEIGHT	REPS	WEIGHT	REPS	WEIGHT

STRETCHING/MOBILITY

ACTIVITY/MOVE	REPS/TIME	NOTES

HERE'S SALUTING YOU FOR COMPLETING WEEK 3! *Don't forget to watch how all your commitment is adding up by tracking key measures in "See Progress" on pages 10 and 11.*

NUTRITION

		TIME	CALORIES	PROTEIN	CARBS	FAT
BREAKFAST						
SNACK						
LUNCH						
SNACK						
DINNER						
SNACK						
DAILY TOTALS						

WATER (8-OZ SERVINGS)

○ ○ ○ ○ ○ ○ ○ ○ ○ ○ ○ ○ ○ ○ ○ ○

SUPPLEMENT	AMOUNT
_____	_____
_____	_____
_____	_____
_____	_____
_____	_____

SLEEP

Lights Out _____

Wake Up _____

Quality:

① ② ③ ④ ⑤
⑥ ⑦ ⑧ ⑨ ⑩

RATE YOUR DAY
On track with goals?

| 10% | 20% | 30% | 40% | 50% | 60% | 70% | 80% | 90% | 100% |

MAP IT

FITNESS

	CARDIO	STRENGTH	STRETCHING/ MOBILITY
DAY 1			
DAY 2			
DAY 3			
DAY 4			
DAY 5			
DAY 6			
DAY 7			

NOTES

NUTRITION

	BREAKFAST	LUNCH	DINNER	SNACKS
DAY 1				
DAY 2				
DAY 3				
DAY 4				
DAY 5				
DAY 6				
DAY 7				

NOTES

_____
_____
_____
_____

TRACK IT

DAY 1

Day of the Week/Date _____

TODAY'S FOCUS

☐ Arms ☐ Legs ☐ Core ☐ Chest ☐ Back ☐ Balance ☐ Flexibility ☐ Total-Body Conditioning

CARDIO

ACTIVITY	MINUTES	LEVEL/SPEED/INTENSITY	HEART RATE	CALORIES BURNED	NOTES

STRENGTH

EXERCISE	SET 1		SET 2		SET 3		SET 4		SET 5	
	REPS	WEIGHT	REPS	WEIGHT	REPS	WEIGHT	REPS	WEIGHT	REPS	WEIGHT

STRETCHING/MOBILITY

ACTIVITY/MOVE	REPS/TIME	NOTES

LET YOUR BUTT SAVE YOUR BACK. *One step can protect your back and make certain strength exercises feel easier. Whenever you're lifting weights over your head, squeeze your butt muscles right before you lift.*

NUTRITION

		TIME	CALORIES	PROTEIN	CARBS	FAT
BREAKFAST						
SNACK						
LUNCH						
SNACK						
DINNER						
SNACK						
DAILY TOTALS						

WATER (8-OZ SERVINGS)

○ ○ ○ ○ ○ ○ ○ ○ ○ ○ ○ ○ ○ ○ ○ ○

SUPPLEMENT	AMOUNT
_____	_____
_____	_____
_____	_____
_____	_____
_____	_____

SLEEP

Lights Out _____

Wake Up _____

Quality:

① ② ③ ④ ⑤
⑥ ⑦ ⑧ ⑨ ⑩

RATE YOUR DAY
On track with goals?

| 10% | 20% | 30% | 40% | 50% | 60% | 70% | 80% | 90% | 100% |

— — TRACK IT — —

DAY 2

Day of the Week/Date _____

TODAY'S FOCUS

☐ Arms   ☐ Legs   ☐ Core   ☐ Chest   ☐ Back   ☐ Balance   ☐ Flexibility   ☐ Total-Body Conditioning

CARDIO

ACTIVITY	MINUTES	LEVEL/SPEED/INTENSITY	HEART RATE	CALORIES BURNED	NOTES

STRENGTH

EXERCISE	SET 1		SET 2		SET 3		SET 4		SET 5	
	REPS	WEIGHT	REPS	WEIGHT	REPS	WEIGHT	REPS	WEIGHT	REPS	WEIGHT

STRETCHING/MOBILITY

ACTIVITY/MOVE	REPS/TIME	NOTES

DON'T SABOTAGE THAT SIX-PACK. *Your abs are muscles, too, so they need a rest between workouts. It's in that process of repairing from microscopic tears that muscles get stronger. Vary the muscles you're working.*

NUTRITION

		TIME	CALORIES	PROTEIN	CARBS	FAT
BREAKFAST						
SNACK						
LUNCH						
SNACK						
DINNER						
SNACK						
DAILY TOTALS						

WATER (8-OZ SERVINGS)

○ ○ ○ ○ ○ ○ ○ ○ ○ ○ ○ ○ ○ ○ ○

SUPPLEMENT	AMOUNT
_____	_____
_____	_____
_____	_____
_____	_____
_____	_____

SLEEP

Lights Out _____

Wake Up _____

Quality:

① ② ③ ④ ⑤
⑥ ⑦ ⑧ ⑨ ⑩

RATE YOUR DAY
On track with goals?

10%	20%	30%	40%	50%	60%	70%	80%	90%	100%

DAY 3

Day of the Week/Date _____

TODAY'S FOCUS

☐ Arms ☐ Legs ☐ Core ☐ Chest ☐ Back ☐ Balance ☐ Flexibility ☐ Total-Body Conditioning

CARDIO

ACTIVITY	MINUTES	LEVEL/SPEED/INTENSITY	HEART RATE	CALORIES BURNED	NOTES

STRENGTH

EXERCISE	SET 1		SET 2		SET 3		SET 4		SET 5	
	REPS	WEIGHT	REPS	WEIGHT	REPS	WEIGHT	REPS	WEIGHT	REPS	WEIGHT

STRETCHING/MOBILITY

ACTIVITY/MOVE	REPS/TIME	NOTES

DO IT FOR YOU. *"The real person you are is revealed in the moments when you're certain no other person is watching. When no one is watching, you are driven by what you expect of yourself."* —*Ralph S. Marston Jr.*

NUTRITION

		TIME	CALORIES	PROTEIN	CARBS	FAT
BREAKFAST						
SNACK						
LUNCH						
SNACK						
DINNER						
SNACK						
DAILY TOTALS						

WATER (8-OZ SERVINGS)

○ ○ ○ ○ ○ ○ ○ ○ ○ ○ ○ ○ ○ ○ ○

SUPPLEMENT	AMOUNT
_____	_____
_____	_____
_____	_____
_____	_____
_____	_____

SLEEP

Lights Out _____

Wake Up _____

Quality:

① ② ③ ④ ⑤
⑥ ⑦ ⑧ ⑨ ⑩

RATE YOUR DAY
On track with goals?

| 10% | 20% | 30% | 40% | 50% | 60% | 70% | 80% | 90% | 100% |

TRACK IT

DAY 4

Day of the Week/Date _____

TODAY'S FOCUS

☐ Arms ☐ Legs ☐ Core ☐ Chest ☐ Back ☐ Balance ☐ Flexibility ☐ Total-Body Conditioning

CARDIO

ACTIVITY	MINUTES	LEVEL/SPEED/ INTENSITY	HEART RATE	CALORIES BURNED	NOTES

STRENGTH

EXERCISE	SET 1		SET 2		SET 3		SET 4		SET 5	
	REPS	WEIGHT	REPS	WEIGHT	REPS	WEIGHT	REPS	WEIGHT	REPS	WEIGHT

STRETCHING/MOBILITY

ACTIVITY/MOVE	REPS/TIME	NOTES

PICK A PROTEIN, NOT CANDY BAR. *For maximum benefits to build muscle, look for a bar with at least 20 grams of protein, 300 calories or fewer, 15 grams of fat or less, and at least 5 grams of fiber.*

NUTRITION

	TIME	CALORIES	PROTEIN	CARBS	FAT
BREAKFAST					
SNACK					
LUNCH					
SNACK					
DINNER					
SNACK					
DAILY TOTALS					

WATER (8-OZ SERVINGS)

○ ○ ○ ○ ○ ○ ○ ○ ○ ○ ○ ○ ○ ○ ○ ○

SUPPLEMENT	AMOUNT
_____	_____
_____	_____
_____	_____
_____	_____
_____	_____

SLEEP

Lights Out _____

Wake Up _____

Quality:

① ② ③ ④ ⑤
⑥ ⑦ ⑧ ⑨ ⑩

RATE YOUR DAY

On track with goals?

10%   20%   30%   40%   50%   60%   70%   80%   90%   100%

DAY 5

Day of the Week/Date _____

TODAY'S FOCUS

☐ Arms ☐ Legs ☐ Core ☐ Chest ☐ Back ☐ Balance ☐ Flexibility ☐ Total-Body Conditioning

CARDIO

ACTIVITY	MINUTES	LEVEL/SPEED/INTENSITY	HEART RATE	CALORIES BURNED	NOTES

STRENGTH

EXERCISE	SET 1		SET 2		SET 3		SET 4		SET 5	
	REPS	WEIGHT	REPS	WEIGHT	REPS	WEIGHT	REPS	WEIGHT	REPS	WEIGHT

STRETCHING/MOBILITY

ACTIVITY/MOVE	REPS/TIME	NOTES

GO AHEAD AND GRUNT. *Researchers found that people who grunted were able to use more force when squeezing a hand grip. Try grunting or exhaling forcefully during your workout.*

NUTRITION

	TIME	CALORIES	PROTEIN	CARBS	FAT
BREAKFAST					
SNACK					
LUNCH					
SNACK					
DINNER					
SNACK					
DAILY TOTALS					

WATER (8-OZ SERVINGS)
○ ○ ○ ○ ○ ○ ○ ○ ○ ○ ○ ○ ○ ○ ○ ○

SUPPLEMENT   **AMOUNT**

_____ | _____
_____ | _____
_____ | _____
_____ | _____
_____ | _____

SLEEP

Lights Out _____

Wake Up _____

Quality:

① ② ③ ④ ⑤
⑥ ⑦ ⑧ ⑨ ⑩

RATE YOUR DAY
On track with goals?

10%   20%   30%   40%   50%   60%   70%   80%   90%   100%

TRACK IT

DAY 6

Day of the Week/Date _____

TODAY'S FOCUS

☐ Arms ☐ Legs ☐ Core ☐ Chest ☐ Back ☐ Balance ☐ Flexibility ☐ Total-Body Conditioning

CARDIO

ACTIVITY	MINUTES	LEVEL/SPEED/INTENSITY	HEART RATE	CALORIES BURNED	NOTES

STRENGTH

EXERCISE	SET 1		SET 2		SET 3		SET 4		SET 5	
	REPS	WEIGHT	REPS	WEIGHT	REPS	WEIGHT	REPS	WEIGHT	REPS	WEIGHT

STRETCHING/MOBILITY

ACTIVITY/MOVE	REPS/TIME	NOTES

STAY TOUGH.

"Never excuse yourself. Never pity yourself. Be a hard master to yourself—and be lenient to everybody else." —*Henry Ward Beecher*

NUTRITION

		TIME	CALORIES	PROTEIN	CARBS	FAT
BREAKFAST						
SNACK						
LUNCH						
SNACK						
DINNER						
SNACK						
DAILY TOTALS						

WATER (8-OZ SERVINGS)

○ ○ ○ ○ ○ ○ ○ ○ ○ ○ ○ ○ ○ ○ ○ ○

SUPPLEMENT	AMOUNT
_____	_____
_____	_____
_____	_____
_____	_____
_____	_____

SLEEP

Lights Out _____

Wake Up _____

Quality:

① ② ③ ④ ⑤
⑥ ⑦ ⑧ ⑨ ⑩

RATE YOUR DAY

On track with goals?

| 10% | 20% | 30% | 40% | 50% | 60% | 70% | 80% | 90% | 100% |

TRACK IT

DAY 7

Day of the Week/Date _____

TODAY'S FOCUS

☐ Arms ☐ Legs ☐ Core ☐ Chest ☐ Back ☐ Balance ☐ Flexibility ☐ Total-Body Conditioning

CARDIO

ACTIVITY	MINUTES	LEVEL/SPEED/ INTENSITY	HEART RATE	CALORIES BURNED	NOTES

STRENGTH

EXERCISE	SET 1		SET 2		SET 3		SET 4		SET 5	
	REPS	WEIGHT	REPS	WEIGHT	REPS	WEIGHT	REPS	WEIGHT	REPS	WEIGHT

STRETCHING/MOBILITY

ACTIVITY/MOVE	REPS/TIME	NOTES

TIME TO CHECK IN! *Note your numbers at the end of this week in "See Progress" on pages 10 and 11. Any other changes—improvement in a sport, an activity that feels easier? Jot those down, too.*

NUTRITION

		TIME	CALORIES	PROTEIN	CARBS	FAT
BREAKFAST						
SNACK						
LUNCH						
SNACK						
DINNER						
SNACK						
DAILY TOTALS						

WATER (8-OZ SERVINGS)

○ ○ ○ ○ ○ ○ ○ ○ ○ ○ ○ ○ ○ ○ ○

SUPPLEMENT	AMOUNT
_____	_____
_____	_____
_____	_____
_____	_____
_____	_____

SLEEP

Lights Out _____

Wake Up _____

Quality:

① ② ③ ④ ⑤
⑥ ⑦ ⑧ ⑨ ⑩

RATE YOUR DAY

On track with goals?

| 10% | 20% | 30% | 40% | 50% | 60% | 70% | 80% | 90% | 100% |

MAP IT

FITNESS

	CARDIO	STRENGTH	STRETCHING/ MOBILITY
DAY 1			
DAY 2			
DAY 3			
DAY 4			
DAY 5			
DAY 6			
DAY 7			

NOTES

NUTRITION

	BREAKFAST	LUNCH	DINNER	SNACKS
DAY 1				
DAY 2				
DAY 3				
DAY 4				
DAY 5				
DAY 6				
DAY 7				

NOTES

_____
_____
_____
_____

TRACK IT

DAY 1

Day of the Week/Date _____

TODAY'S FOCUS

☐ Arms ☐ Legs ☐ Core ☐ Chest ☐ Back ☐ Balance ☐ Flexibility ☐ Total-Body Conditioning

CARDIO

ACTIVITY	MINUTES	LEVEL/SPEED/INTENSITY	HEART RATE	CALORIES BURNED	NOTES

STRENGTH

EXERCISE	SET 1		SET 2		SET 3		SET 4		SET 5	
	REPS	WEIGHT	REPS	WEIGHT	REPS	WEIGHT	REPS	WEIGHT	REPS	WEIGHT

STRETCHING/MOBILITY

ACTIVITY/MOVE	REPS/TIME	NOTES

MAKE A FRIENDLY WAGER. *Challenge a rival to a contest—whether it's a time for running a mile or amount of weight bench-pressed. Research has found that competition can drive motivation.*

NUTRITION

		TIME	CALORIES	PROTEIN	CARBS	FAT
BREAKFAST						
SNACK						
LUNCH						
SNACK						
DINNER						
SNACK						
	DAILY TOTALS					

WATER (8-OZ SERVINGS)

○ ○ ○ ○ ○ ○ ○ ○ ○ ○ ○ ○ ○ ○ ○ ○

SUPPLEMENT	AMOUNT
_____	_____
_____	_____
_____	_____
_____	_____
_____	_____

SLEEP

Lights Out _____

Wake Up _____

Quality:

① ② ③ ④ ⑤
⑥ ⑦ ⑧ ⑨ ⑩

RATE YOUR DAY
On track with goals?

| 10% | 20% | 30% | 40% | 50% | 60% | 70% | 80% | 90% | 100% |

DAY 2

Day of the Week/Date _____

TODAY'S FOCUS

☐ Arms ☐ Legs ☐ Core ☐ Chest ☐ Back ☐ Balance ☐ Flexibility ☐ Total-Body Conditioning

CARDIO

ACTIVITY	MINUTES	LEVEL/SPEED/INTENSITY	HEART RATE	CALORIES BURNED	NOTES

STRENGTH

EXERCISE	SET 1		SET 2		SET 3		SET 4		SET 5	
	REPS	WEIGHT	REPS	WEIGHT	REPS	WEIGHT	REPS	WEIGHT	REPS	WEIGHT

STRETCHING/MOBILITY

ACTIVITY/MOVE	REPS/TIME	NOTES

BUILD MUSCLE WITH OMEGA-3S. *These good fats decrease muscle breakdown and help your body use protein better to boost muscle. You can find omega-3s in fish, avocados, nuts, leafy greens, and supplements.*

NUTRITION

	TIME	CALORIES	PROTEIN	CARBS	FAT
BREAKFAST					
SNACK					
LUNCH					
SNACK					
DINNER					
SNACK					
DAILY TOTALS					

WATER (8-OZ SERVINGS)

○ ○ ○ ○ ○ ○ ○ ○ ○ ○ ○ ○ ○ ○ ○

SUPPLEMENT   **AMOUNT**

_____ | _____
_____ | _____
_____ | _____
_____ | _____
_____ | _____

SLEEP

Lights Out _____

Wake Up _____

Quality:

① ② ③ ④ ⑤
⑥ ⑦ ⑧ ⑨ ⑩

RATE YOUR DAY

On track with goals?

| 10% | 20% | 30% | 40% | 50% | 60% | 70% | 80% | 90% | 100% |

TRACK IT

DAY 3

Day of the Week/Date _____

TODAY'S FOCUS

☐ Arms ☐ Legs ☐ Core ☐ Chest ☐ Back ☐ Balance ☐ Flexibility ☐ Total-Body Conditioning

CARDIO

ACTIVITY	MINUTES	LEVEL/SPEED/INTENSITY	HEART RATE	CALORIES BURNED	NOTES

STRENGTH

EXERCISE	SET 1		SET 2		SET 3		SET 4		SET 5	
	REPS	WEIGHT	REPS	WEIGHT	REPS	WEIGHT	REPS	WEIGHT	REPS	WEIGHT

STRETCHING/MOBILITY

ACTIVITY/MOVE	REPS/TIME	NOTES

NO LIMITS.

"Do just once what others say you can't do, and you will never pay attention to their limitations again." —James R. Cook

NUTRITION

		TIME	CALORIES	PROTEIN	CARBS	FAT
BREAKFAST						
SNACK						
LUNCH						
SNACK						
DINNER						
SNACK						
DAILY TOTALS						

WATER (8-OZ SERVINGS)

○ ○ ○ ○ ○ ○ ○ ○ ○ ○ ○ ○ ○ ○ ○ ○

SUPPLEMENT	AMOUNT
_____	_____
_____	_____
_____	_____
_____	_____
_____	_____

SLEEP

Lights Out _____

Wake Up _____

Quality:

① ② ③ ④ ⑤
⑥ ⑦ ⑧ ⑨ ⑩

RATE YOUR DAY

On track with goals?

| 10% | 20% | 30% | 40% | 50% | 60% | 70% | 80% | 90% | 100% |

TRACK IT

DAY 4

Day of the Week/Date _____

TODAY'S FOCUS

☐ Arms ☐ Legs ☐ Core ☐ Chest ☐ Back ☐ Balance ☐ Flexibility ☐ Total-Body Conditioning

CARDIO

ACTIVITY	MINUTES	LEVEL/SPEED/INTENSITY	HEART RATE	CALORIES BURNED	NOTES

STRENGTH

EXERCISE	SET 1		SET 2		SET 3		SET 4		SET 5	
	REPS	WEIGHT	REPS	WEIGHT	REPS	WEIGHT	REPS	WEIGHT	REPS	WEIGHT

STRETCHING/MOBILITY

ACTIVITY/MOVE	REPS/TIME	NOTES

DIG IN THOSE HEELS. *When doing standing leg exercises, concentrate on your heels and driving them into the ground. This technique makes the move feel easier, activates large muscles, and keeps your form stable.*

NUTRITION

		TIME	CALORIES	PROTEIN	CARBS	FAT
BREAKFAST						
SNACK						
LUNCH						
SNACK						
DINNER						
SNACK						
DAILY TOTALS						

WATER (8-OZ SERVINGS)

○ ○ ○ ○ ○ ○ ○ ○ ○ ○ ○ ○ ○ ○ ○ ○

SUPPLEMENT	AMOUNT
_____	_____
_____	_____
_____	_____
_____	_____
_____	_____

SLEEP

Lights Out _____

Wake Up _____

Quality:

① ② ③ ④ ⑤
⑥ ⑦ ⑧ ⑨ ⑩

RATE YOUR DAY

On track with goals?

| 10% | 20% | 30% | 40% | 50% | 60% | 70% | 80% | 90% | 100% |

DAY 5

Day of the Week/Date _____

TODAY'S FOCUS

☐ Arms ☐ Legs ☐ Core ☐ Chest ☐ Back ☐ Balance ☐ Flexibility ☐ Total-Body Conditioning

CARDIO

ACTIVITY	MINUTES	LEVEL/SPEED/INTENSITY	HEART RATE	CALORIES BURNED	NOTES

STRENGTH

EXERCISE	SET 1		SET 2		SET 3		SET 4		SET 5	
	REPS	WEIGHT	REPS	WEIGHT	REPS	WEIGHT	REPS	WEIGHT	REPS	WEIGHT

STRETCHING/MOBILITY

ACTIVITY/MOVE	REPS/TIME	NOTES

FOCUS ON THE GOAL. *Researchers found that people who looked straight ahead while walking moved 23 percent faster than those who let their eyes take in the surrounding sights. They also said the workout felt easier.*

NUTRITION

	TIME	CALORIES	PROTEIN	CARBS	FAT
BREAKFAST					
SNACK					
LUNCH					
SNACK					
DINNER					
SNACK					
DAILY TOTALS					

WATER (8-OZ SERVINGS)

○ ○ ○ ○ ○ ○ ○ ○ ○ ○ ○ ○ ○ ○ ○

SUPPLEMENT	AMOUNT
_____	_____
_____	_____
_____	_____
_____	_____
_____	_____

SLEEP

Lights Out _____

Wake Up _____

Quality:

① ② ③ ④ ⑤
⑥ ⑦ ⑧ ⑨ ⑩

RATE YOUR DAY

On track with goals?

10%   20%   30%   40%   50%   60%   70%   80%   90%   100%

TRACK IT

DAY 6

Day of the Week/Date _____

TODAY'S FOCUS

☐ Arms   ☐ Legs   ☐ Core   ☐ Chest   ☐ Back   ☐ Balance   ☐ Flexibility   ☐ Total-Body Conditioning

CARDIO

ACTIVITY	MINUTES	LEVEL/SPEED/INTENSITY	HEART RATE	CALORIES BURNED	NOTES

STRENGTH

EXERCISE	SET 1		SET 2		SET 3		SET 4		SET 5	
	REPS	WEIGHT	REPS	WEIGHT	REPS	WEIGHT	REPS	WEIGHT	REPS	WEIGHT

STRETCHING/MOBILITY

ACTIVITY/MOVE	REPS/TIME	NOTES

MAKE A SMART MOVE.

"No matter how slow you go, you're still lapping everybody on the couch."
—Anonymous

NUTRITION

		TIME	CALORIES	PROTEIN	CARBS	FAT
BREAKFAST						
SNACK						
LUNCH						
SNACK						
DINNER						
SNACK						
	DAILY TOTALS					

WATER (8-OZ SERVINGS)

○ ○ ○ ○ ○ ○ ○ ○ ○ ○ ○ ○ ○ ○ ○ ○

SUPPLEMENT	AMOUNT
_____	_____
_____	_____
_____	_____
_____	_____
_____	_____

SLEEP

Lights Out _____

Wake Up _____

Quality:

① ② ③ ④ ⑤
⑥ ⑦ ⑧ ⑨ ⑩

RATE YOUR DAY
On track with goals?

| 10% | 20% | 30% | 40% | 50% | 60% | 70% | 80% | 90% | 100% |

TRACK IT

DAY 7

Day of the Week/Date _____

TODAY'S FOCUS

☐ Arms ☐ Legs ☐ Core ☐ Chest ☐ Back ☐ Balance ☐ Flexibility ☐ Total-Body Conditioning

CARDIO

ACTIVITY	MINUTES	LEVEL/SPEED/INTENSITY	HEART RATE	CALORIES BURNED	NOTES

STRENGTH

EXERCISE	SET 1		SET 2		SET 3		SET 4		SET 5	
	REPS	WEIGHT	REPS	WEIGHT	REPS	WEIGHT	REPS	WEIGHT	REPS	WEIGHT

STRETCHING/MOBILITY

ACTIVITY/MOVE	REPS/TIME	NOTES

SEEING PROGRESS? *Hit up pages 10 and 11 to make sure you have a record. For many goals, you'll also start seeing the progress in the mirror and in the way your clothing fits—note that, too.*

NUTRITION

	TIME	CALORIES	PROTEIN	CARBS	FAT
BREAKFAST					
SNACK					
LUNCH					
SNACK					
DINNER					
SNACK					
DAILY TOTALS					

WATER (8-OZ SERVINGS)

○ ○ ○ ○ ○ ○ ○ ○ ○ ○ ○ ○ ○ ○ ○ ○

SUPPLEMENT   **AMOUNT**

_____ | _____
_____ | _____
_____ | _____
_____ | _____
_____ | _____

SLEEP

Lights Out _____

Wake Up _____

Quality:

① ② ③ ④ ⑤
⑥ ⑦ ⑧ ⑨ ⑩

RATE YOUR DAY
On track with goals?

| 10% | 20% | 30% | 40% | 50% | 60% | 70% | 80% | 90% | 100% |

MAP IT

FITNESS

	CARDIO	STRENGTH	STRETCHING/ MOBILITY
DAY 1			
DAY 2			
DAY 3			
DAY 4			
DAY 5			
DAY 6			
DAY 7			

NOTES

_____
_____
_____
_____

NUTRITION

	BREAKFAST	LUNCH	DINNER	SNACKS
DAY 1				
DAY 2				
DAY 3				
DAY 4				
DAY 5				
DAY 6				
DAY 7				

NOTES

_____
_____
_____
_____

TRACK IT

DAY 1

Day of the Week/Date _____

TODAY'S FOCUS

☐ Arms ☐ Legs ☐ Core ☐ Chest ☐ Back ☐ Balance ☐ Flexibility ☐ Total-Body Conditioning

CARDIO

ACTIVITY	MINUTES	LEVEL/SPEED/INTENSITY	HEART RATE	CALORIES BURNED	NOTES

STRENGTH

EXERCISE	SET 1		SET 2		SET 3		SET 4		SET 5	
	REPS	WEIGHT	REPS	WEIGHT	REPS	WEIGHT	REPS	WEIGHT	REPS	WEIGHT

STRETCHING/MOBILITY

ACTIVITY/MOVE	REPS/TIME	NOTES

PICK IT UP WITH A PLAYLIST. *Studies have shown that people who exercise while listening to music will do so longer and more intensely than people who exercise without music. Turn it up, and push out those last reps!*

NUTRITION

		TIME	CALORIES	PROTEIN	CARBS	FAT
BREAKFAST						
SNACK						
LUNCH						
SNACK						
DINNER						
SNACK						
	DAILY TOTALS					

WATER (8-OZ SERVINGS)

○ ○ ○ ○ ○ ○ ○ ○ ○ ○ ○ ○ ○ ○ ○

SUPPLEMENT	AMOUNT
_____	_____
_____	_____
_____	_____
_____	_____
_____	_____

SLEEP

Lights Out _____

Wake Up _____

Quality:

(1) (2) (3) (4) (5)

(6) (7) (8) (9) (10)

RATE YOUR DAY
On track with goals?

| 10% | 20% | 30% | 40% | 50% | 60% | 70% | 80% | 90% | 100% |

DAY 2

Day of the Week/Date _____

TODAY'S FOCUS

☐ Arms   ☐ Legs   ☐ Core   ☐ Chest   ☐ Back   ☐ Balance   ☐ Flexibility   ☐ Total-Body Conditioning

CARDIO

ACTIVITY	MINUTES	LEVEL/SPEED/ INTENSITY	HEART RATE	CALORIES BURNED	NOTES

STRENGTH

EXERCISE	SET 1		SET 2		SET 3		SET 4		SET 5	
	REPS	WEIGHT	REPS	WEIGHT	REPS	WEIGHT	REPS	WEIGHT	REPS	WEIGHT

STRETCHING/MOBILITY

ACTIVITY/MOVE	REPS/TIME	NOTES

BEST TIME TO WORK OUT? *Some say it's morning, before anything gets in the way. Others say they don't come alive until the afternoon. What does the research say? Any workout will feel easier during your own peak hours.*

NUTRITION

		TIME	CALORIES	PROTEIN	CARBS	FAT
BREAKFAST						
SNACK						
LUNCH						
SNACK						
DINNER						
SNACK						
DAILY TOTALS						

WATER (8-OZ SERVINGS)

○ ○ ○ ○ ○ ○ ○ ○ ○ ○ ○ ○ ○ ○ ○

SUPPLEMENT	AMOUNT
_____	_____
_____	_____
_____	_____
_____	_____
_____	_____

SLEEP

Lights Out _____

Wake Up _____

Quality:

① ② ③ ④ ⑤
⑥ ⑦ ⑧ ⑨ ⑩

RATE YOUR DAY
On track with goals?

10%	20%	30%	40%	50%	60%	70%	80%	90%	100%

DAY 3

Day of the Week/Date _____

TODAY'S FOCUS

☐ Arms ☐ Legs ☐ Core ☐ Chest ☐ Back ☐ Balance ☐ Flexibility ☐ Total-Body Conditioning

CARDIO

ACTIVITY	MINUTES	LEVEL/SPEED/INTENSITY	HEART RATE	CALORIES BURNED	NOTES

STRENGTH

EXERCISE	SET 1		SET 2		SET 3		SET 4		SET 5	
	REPS	WEIGHT	REPS	WEIGHT	REPS	WEIGHT	REPS	WEIGHT	REPS	WEIGHT

STRETCHING/MOBILITY

ACTIVITY/MOVE	REPS/TIME	NOTES

MOVE OUT OF THE COMFORT ZONE. *"Action breeds confidence and courage. If you want to conquer fear, do not sit home and think about it. Go out and get busy." —Dale Carnegie*

NUTRITION

		TIME	CALORIES	PROTEIN	CARBS	FAT
BREAKFAST						
SNACK						
LUNCH						
SNACK						
DINNER						
SNACK						
DAILY TOTALS						

WATER (8-OZ SERVINGS)

○ ○ ○ ○ ○ ○ ○ ○ ○ ○ ○ ○ ○ ○ ○

SUPPLEMENT   **AMOUNT**

_____ | _____

_____ | _____

_____ | _____

_____ | _____

_____ | _____

SLEEP

Lights Out _____

Wake Up _____

Quality:

① ② ③ ④ ⑤

⑥ ⑦ ⑧ ⑨ ⑩

RATE YOUR DAY

On track with goals?

10% 20% 30% 40% 50% 60% 70% 80% 90% 100%

TRACK IT

DAY 4

Day of the Week/Date _____

TODAY'S FOCUS

☐ Arms ☐ Legs ☐ Core ☐ Chest ☐ Back ☐ Balance ☐ Flexibility ☐ Total-Body Conditioning

CARDIO

ACTIVITY	MINUTES	LEVEL/SPEED/INTENSITY	HEART RATE	CALORIES BURNED	NOTES

STRENGTH

EXERCISE	SET 1		SET 2		SET 3		SET 4		SET 5	
	REPS	WEIGHT	REPS	WEIGHT	REPS	WEIGHT	REPS	WEIGHT	REPS	WEIGHT

STRETCHING/MOBILITY

ACTIVITY/MOVE	REPS/TIME	NOTES

CHECK YOUR SLEEP. *Your muscles need sleep to really show up at the gym, on your run, or on the bike. To get more sleep, try turning off electronics and winding down sooner (without alcohol) tonight.*

NUTRITION

	TIME	CALORIES	PROTEIN	CARBS	FAT
BREAKFAST					
SNACK					
LUNCH					
SNACK					
DINNER					
SNACK					
DAILY TOTALS					

WATER (8-OZ SERVINGS)

○ ○ ○ ○ ○ ○ ○ ○ ○ ○ ○ ○ ○ ○ ○

SUPPLEMENT   **AMOUNT**

_____ _____

_____ _____

_____ _____

_____ _____

_____ _____

SLEEP

Lights Out _____

Wake Up _____

Quality:

① ② ③ ④ ⑤
⑥ ⑦ ⑧ ⑨ ⑩

RATE YOUR DAY
On track with goals?

| 10% | 20% | 30% | 40% | 50% | 60% | 70% | 80% | 90% | 100% |

DAY 5

Day of the Week/Date _____

TODAY'S FOCUS

☐ Arms ☐ Legs ☐ Core ☐ Chest ☐ Back ☐ Balance ☐ Flexibility ☐ Total-Body Conditioning

CARDIO

ACTIVITY	MINUTES	LEVEL/SPEED/INTENSITY	HEART RATE	CALORIES BURNED	NOTES

STRENGTH

EXERCISE	SET 1		SET 2		SET 3		SET 4		SET 5	
	REPS	WEIGHT	REPS	WEIGHT	REPS	WEIGHT	REPS	WEIGHT	REPS	WEIGHT

STRETCHING/MOBILITY

ACTIVITY/MOVE	REPS/TIME	NOTES

TEAM UP CARDIO AND STRENGTH. *Add intervals of jumping rope or burpees between strength sets to create a muscle-building, metabolism-revving workout—great for days when time is short.*

NUTRITION

		TIME	CALORIES	PROTEIN	CARBS	FAT
BREAKFAST						
SNACK						
LUNCH						
SNACK						
DINNER						
SNACK						
DAILY TOTALS						

WATER (8-OZ SERVINGS)

○ ○ ○ ○ ○ ○ ○ ○ ○ ○ ○ ○ ○ ○ ○ ○

SUPPLEMENT   **AMOUNT**

_____ | _____
_____ | _____
_____ | _____
_____ | _____
_____ | _____

SLEEP

Lights Out _____

Wake Up _____

Quality:

① ② ③ ④ ⑤
⑥ ⑦ ⑧ ⑨ ⑩

RATE YOUR DAY

On track with goals?

| 10% | 20% | 30% | 40% | 50% | 60% | 70% | 80% | 90% | 100% |

DAY 6

Day of the Week/Date _____

TODAY'S FOCUS

☐ Arms ☐ Legs ☐ Core ☐ Chest ☐ Back ☐ Balance ☐ Flexibility ☐ Total-Body Conditioning

CARDIO

ACTIVITY	MINUTES	LEVEL/SPEED/INTENSITY	HEART RATE	CALORIES BURNED	NOTES

STRENGTH

EXERCISE	SET 1		SET 2		SET 3		SET 4		SET 5	
	REPS	WEIGHT	REPS	WEIGHT	REPS	WEIGHT	REPS	WEIGHT	REPS	WEIGHT

STRETCHING/MOBILITY

ACTIVITY/MOVE	REPS/TIME	NOTES

GO FOR BETTER THAN GOOD.

"Great things come from hard work and perseverance. No excuses."
—Kobe Bryant

NUTRITION

		TIME	CALORIES	PROTEIN	CARBS	FAT
BREAKFAST						
SNACK						
LUNCH						
SNACK						
DINNER						
SNACK						
DAILY TOTALS						

WATER (8-OZ SERVINGS)

○ ○ ○ ○ ○ ○ ○ ○ ○ ○ ○ ○ ○ ○

SUPPLEMENT	AMOUNT
_____	_____
_____	_____
_____	_____
_____	_____
_____	_____

SLEEP

Lights Out _____

Wake Up _____

Quality:

① ② ③ ④ ⑤
⑥ ⑦ ⑧ ⑨ ⑩

RATE YOUR DAY

On track with goals?

| 10% | 20% | 30% | 40% | 50% | 60% | 70% | 80% | 90% | 100% |

DAY 7

Day of the Week/Date _____

TODAY'S FOCUS

☐ Arms ☐ Legs ☐ Core ☐ Chest ☐ Back ☐ Balance ☐ Flexibility ☐ Total-Body Conditioning

CARDIO

ACTIVITY	MINUTES	LEVEL/SPEED/INTENSITY	HEART RATE	CALORIES BURNED	NOTES

STRENGTH

EXERCISE	SET 1		SET 2		SET 3		SET 4		SET 5	
	REPS	WEIGHT	REPS	WEIGHT	REPS	WEIGHT	REPS	WEIGHT	REPS	WEIGHT

STRETCHING/MOBILITY

ACTIVITY/MOVE	REPS/TIME	NOTES

ALMOST HALFWAY TO 90 DAYS! *Today's the day to check in with your numbers on pages 10 and 11. This week, consider sharing your goals and progress with a friend for even more accountability.*

NUTRITION

		TIME	CALORIES	PROTEIN	CARBS	FAT
BREAKFAST						
SNACK						
LUNCH						
SNACK						
DINNER						
SNACK						
DAILY TOTALS						

WATER (8-OZ SERVINGS)

○ ○ ○ ○ ○ ○ ○ ○ ○ ○ ○ ○ ○ ○ ○

SUPPLEMENT	AMOUNT
_____	_____
_____	_____
_____	_____
_____	_____
_____	_____

SLEEP

Lights Out _____

Wake Up _____

Quality:

① ② ③ ④ ⑤
⑥ ⑦ ⑧ ⑨ ⑩

RATE YOUR DAY
On track with goals?

| 10% | 20% | 30% | 40% | 50% | 60% | 70% | 80% | 90% | 100% |

FITNESS

	CARDIO	STRENGTH	STRETCHING/ MOBILITY
DAY 1			
DAY 2			
DAY 3			
DAY 4			
DAY 5			
DAY 6			
DAY 7			

NOTES

NUTRITION

	BREAKFAST	LUNCH	DINNER	SNACKS
DAY 1				
DAY 2				
DAY 3				
DAY 4				
DAY 5				
DAY 6				
DAY 7				

NOTES

DAY 1

Day of the Week/Date _____

TODAY'S FOCUS

☐ Arms ☐ Legs ☐ Core ☐ Chest ☐ Back ☐ Balance ☐ Flexibility ☐ Total-Body Conditioning

CARDIO

ACTIVITY	MINUTES	LEVEL/SPEED/INTENSITY	HEART RATE	CALORIES BURNED	NOTES

STRENGTH

EXERCISE	SET 1		SET 2		SET 3		SET 4		SET 5	
	REPS	WEIGHT	REPS	WEIGHT	REPS	WEIGHT	REPS	WEIGHT	REPS	WEIGHT

STRETCHING/MOBILITY

ACTIVITY/MOVE	REPS/TIME	NOTES

NEED AN EXTRA CHALLENGE? *Build a little instability into your workout. Exercises that require balance stimulate more muscles than the same exercise done in a stable position. Try one-legged squats or push-ups on a stability ball.*

NUTRITION

		TIME	CALORIES	PROTEIN	CARBS	FAT
BREAKFAST						
SNACK						
LUNCH						
SNACK						
DINNER						
SNACK						
DAILY TOTALS						

WATER (8-OZ SERVINGS)

○ ○ ○ ○ ○ ○ ○ ○ ○ ○ ○ ○ ○ ○ ○ ○

SUPPLEMENT   **AMOUNT**

_____ | _____

_____ | _____

_____ | _____

_____ | _____

_____ | _____

SLEEP

Lights Out _____

Wake Up _____

Quality:

① ② ③ ④ ⑤
⑥ ⑦ ⑧ ⑨ ⑩

RATE YOUR DAY

On track with goals?

| 10% | 20% | 30% | 40% | 50% | 60% | 70% | 80% | 90% | 100% |

DAY 2

Day of the Week/Date _____

TODAY'S FOCUS

☐ Arms ☐ Legs ☐ Core ☐ Chest ☐ Back ☐ Balance ☐ Flexibility ☐ Total-Body Conditioning

CARDIO

ACTIVITY	MINUTES	LEVEL/SPEED/INTENSITY	HEART RATE	CALORIES BURNED	NOTES

STRENGTH

EXERCISE	SET 1		SET 2		SET 3		SET 4		SET 5	
	REPS	WEIGHT	REPS	WEIGHT	REPS	WEIGHT	REPS	WEIGHT	REPS	WEIGHT

STRETCHING/MOBILITY

ACTIVITY/MOVE	REPS/TIME	NOTES

TACKLE WHAT YOU DREAD. *Switch your workout around and do the hardest moves first to give yourself a psychological edge. You'll get them out of the way and end the workout with moves you enjoy and that feel easier.*

NUTRITION

		TIME	CALORIES	PROTEIN	CARBS	FAT
BREAKFAST						
SNACK						
LUNCH						
SNACK						
DINNER						
SNACK						
	DAILY TOTALS					

WATER (8-OZ SERVINGS)

○ ○ ○ ○ ○ ○ ○ ○ ○ ○ ○ ○ ○ ○ ○

SUPPLEMENT	AMOUNT
_____	_____
_____	_____
_____	_____
_____	_____
_____	_____

SLEEP

Lights Out _____

Wake Up _____

Quality:

① ② ③ ④ ⑤
⑥ ⑦ ⑧ ⑨ ⑩

RATE YOUR DAY

On track with goals?

| 10% | 20% | 30% | 40% | 50% | 60% | 70% | 80% | 90% | 100% |

TRACK IT

DAY 3

Day of the Week/Date _____

TODAY'S FOCUS

☐ Arms ☐ Legs ☐ Core ☐ Chest ☐ Back ☐ Balance ☐ Flexibility ☐ Total-Body Conditioning

CARDIO

ACTIVITY	MINUTES	LEVEL/SPEED/INTENSITY	HEART RATE	CALORIES BURNED	NOTES

STRENGTH

EXERCISE	SET 1		SET 2		SET 3		SET 4		SET 5	
	REPS	WEIGHT	REPS	WEIGHT	REPS	WEIGHT	REPS	WEIGHT	REPS	WEIGHT

STRETCHING/MOBILITY

ACTIVITY/MOVE	REPS/TIME	NOTES

HAVE WHAT IT TAKES?

"We all have dreams. But in order to make dreams come into reality, it takes an awful lot of determination, dedication, self-discipline, and effort." —*Jesse Owens*

NUTRITION

		TIME	CALORIES	PROTEIN	CARBS	FAT
BREAKFAST						
SNACK						
LUNCH						
SNACK						
DINNER						
SNACK						
DAILY TOTALS						

WATER (8-OZ SERVINGS)

◯ ◯ ◯ ◯ ◯ ◯ ◯ ◯ ◯ ◯ ◯ ◯ ◯ ◯ ◯

SUPPLEMENT	AMOUNT
_____	_____
_____	_____
_____	_____
_____	_____
_____	_____

SLEEP

Lights Out _____

Wake Up _____

Quality:

① ② ③ ④ ⑤
⑥ ⑦ ⑧ ⑨ ⑩

RATE YOUR DAY

On track with goals?

10%   20%   30%   40%   50%   60%   70%   80%   90%   100%

TRACK IT

DAY 4   Day of the Week/Date _____

TODAY'S FOCUS

☐ Arms ☐ Legs ☐ Core ☐ Chest ☐ Back ☐ Balance ☐ Flexibility ☐ Total-Body Conditioning

CARDIO

ACTIVITY	MINUTES	LEVEL/SPEED/INTENSITY	HEART RATE	CALORIES BURNED	NOTES

STRENGTH

EXERCISE	SET 1		SET 2		SET 3		SET 4		SET 5	
	REPS	WEIGHT	REPS	WEIGHT	REPS	WEIGHT	REPS	WEIGHT	REPS	WEIGHT

STRETCHING/MOBILITY

ACTIVITY/MOVE	REPS/TIME	NOTES

COMMIT TO A MINIMUM. *On days you're not feeling a workout, promise yourself to do just one set or just 10 minutes. Chances are, once you get started, it will seem silly to stop, and you'll finish the workout.*

NUTRITION

		TIME	CALORIES	PROTEIN	CARBS	FAT
BREAKFAST						
SNACK						
LUNCH						
SNACK						
DINNER						
SNACK						
DAILY TOTALS						

WATER (8-OZ SERVINGS)

○ ○ ○ ○ ○ ○ ○ ○ ○ ○ ○ ○ ○ ○

SUPPLEMENT   **AMOUNT**

_____ | _____

_____ | _____

_____ | _____

_____ | _____

_____ | _____

SLEEP

Lights Out _____

Wake Up _____

Quality:

① ② ③ ④ ⑤

⑥ ⑦ ⑧ ⑨ ⑩

RATE YOUR DAY

On track with goals?

10%	20%	30%	40%	50%	60%	70%	80%	90%	100%

TRACK IT

DAY 5

Day of the Week/Date _____

TODAY'S FOCUS

☐ Arms ☐ Legs ☐ Core ☐ Chest ☐ Back ☐ Balance ☐ Flexibility ☐ Total-Body Conditioning

CARDIO

ACTIVITY	MINUTES	LEVEL/SPEED/INTENSITY	HEART RATE	CALORIES BURNED	NOTES

STRENGTH

EXERCISE	SET 1		SET 2		SET 3		SET 4		SET 5	
	REPS	WEIGHT	REPS	WEIGHT	REPS	WEIGHT	REPS	WEIGHT	REPS	WEIGHT

STRETCHING/MOBILITY

ACTIVITY/MOVE	REPS/TIME	NOTES

GET FAST-TWITCH STRONG. *It pays to mix slow, heavy lifts for strength with more explosive movements that target fast-twitch muscle fibers for power. For fast-twitch focus, try kettlebell swings and box jumps.*

NUTRITION

		TIME	CALORIES	PROTEIN	CARBS	FAT
BREAKFAST						
SNACK						
LUNCH						
SNACK						
DINNER						
SNACK						
	DAILY TOTALS					

WATER (8-OZ SERVINGS)

○ ○ ○ ○ ○ ○ ○ ○ ○ ○ ○ ○ ○ ○

SUPPLEMENT	AMOUNT
_____	_____
_____	_____
_____	_____
_____	_____
_____	_____

SLEEP

Lights Out _____

Wake Up _____

Quality:

① ② ③ ④ ⑤
⑥ ⑦ ⑧ ⑨ ⑩

RATE YOUR DAY
On track with goals?

10% 20% 30% 40% 50% 60% 70% 80% 90% 100%

DAY 6

Day of the Week/Date _____

TODAY'S FOCUS

☐ Arms   ☐ Legs   ☐ Core   ☐ Chest   ☐ Back   ☐ Balance   ☐ Flexibility   ☐ Total-Body Conditioning

CARDIO

ACTIVITY	MINUTES	LEVEL/SPEED/INTENSITY	HEART RATE	CALORIES BURNED	NOTES

STRENGTH

EXERCISE	SET 1		SET 2		SET 3		SET 4		SET 5	
	REPS	WEIGHT	REPS	WEIGHT	REPS	WEIGHT	REPS	WEIGHT	REPS	WEIGHT

STRETCHING/MOBILITY

ACTIVITY/MOVE	REPS/TIME	NOTES

CHANGE YOUR LIFE.

"It's not what we do once in a while that shapes our lives. It's what we do consistently." —Tony Robbins

NUTRITION

		TIME	CALORIES	PROTEIN	CARBS	FAT
BREAKFAST						
SNACK						
LUNCH						
SNACK						
DINNER						
SNACK						
DAILY TOTALS						

WATER (8-OZ SERVINGS)

○ ○ ○ ○ ○ ○ ○ ○ ○ ○ ○ ○ ○ ○ ○ ○

SUPPLEMENT	AMOUNT
_____	_____
_____	_____
_____	_____
_____	_____
_____	_____

SLEEP

Lights Out _____

Wake Up _____

Quality:

① ② ③ ④ ⑤
⑥ ⑦ ⑧ ⑨ ⑩

RATE YOUR DAY

On track with goals?

| 10% | 20% | 30% | 40% | 50% | 60% | 70% | 80% | 90% | 100% |

DAY 7

Day of the Week/Date _____

TODAY'S FOCUS

☐ Arms ☐ Legs ☐ Core ☐ Chest ☐ Back ☐ Balance ☐ Flexibility ☐ Total-Body Conditioning

CARDIO

ACTIVITY	MINUTES	LEVEL/SPEED/ INTENSITY	HEART RATE	CALORIES BURNED	NOTES

STRENGTH

EXERCISE	SET 1		SET 2		SET 3		SET 4		SET 5	
	REPS	WEIGHT	REPS	WEIGHT	REPS	WEIGHT	REPS	WEIGHT	REPS	WEIGHT

STRETCHING/MOBILITY

ACTIVITY/MOVE	REPS/TIME	NOTES

DO THE NUMBERS. *It's the end of another workout week and time to head over to "See Progress" on pages 10 and 11. You'll get motivation to head strong into week 8!*

NUTRITION

		TIME	CALORIES	PROTEIN	CARBS	FAT
BREAKFAST						
SNACK						
LUNCH						
SNACK						
DINNER						
SNACK						
DAILY TOTALS						

WATER (8-OZ SERVINGS)

○ ○ ○ ○ ○ ○ ○ ○ ○ ○ ○ ○ ○ ○ ○

SUPPLEMENT	**AMOUNT**
_____	_____
_____	_____
_____	_____
_____	_____
_____	_____

SLEEP

Lights Out _____

Wake Up _____

Quality:

① ② ③ ④ ⑤
⑥ ⑦ ⑧ ⑨ ⑩

RATE YOUR DAY
On track with goals?

| 10% | 20% | 30% | 40% | 50% | 60% | 70% | 80% | 90% | 100% |

MAP IT

FITNESS

	CARDIO	STRENGTH	STRETCHING/ MOBILITY
DAY 1			
DAY 2			
DAY 3			
DAY 4			
DAY 5			
DAY 6			
DAY 7			

NOTES

NUTRITION

	BREAKFAST	LUNCH	DINNER	SNACKS
DAY 1				
DAY 2				
DAY 3				
DAY 4				
DAY 5				
DAY 6				
DAY 7				

NOTES

TRACK IT

DAY 1

Day of the Week/Date _____

TODAY'S FOCUS

☐ Arms ☐ Legs ☐ Core ☐ Chest ☐ Back ☐ Balance ☐ Flexibility ☐ Total-Body Conditioning

CARDIO

ACTIVITY	MINUTES	LEVEL/SPEED/ INTENSITY	HEART RATE	CALORIES BURNED	NOTES

STRENGTH

EXERCISE	SET 1		SET 2		SET 3		SET 4		SET 5	
	REPS	WEIGHT	REPS	WEIGHT	REPS	WEIGHT	REPS	WEIGHT	REPS	WEIGHT

STRETCHING/MOBILITY

ACTIVITY/MOVE	REPS/TIME	NOTES

BRAG ON SOCIAL MEDIA. *Don't think twice about sharing progress. It'll give you a boost to pat yourself on the back. Plus, research has found that posting your fitness goals and accomplishments can inspire others. Win-win.*

NUTRITION

		TIME	CALORIES	PROTEIN	CARBS	FAT
BREAKFAST						
SNACK						
LUNCH						
SNACK						
DINNER						
SNACK						
DAILY TOTALS						

WATER (8-OZ SERVINGS)

○ ○ ○ ○ ○ ○ ○ ○ ○ ○ ○ ○ ○ ○ ○

SUPPLEMENT	**AMOUNT**
_____	_____
_____	_____
_____	_____
_____	_____
_____	_____

SLEEP

Lights Out _____

Wake Up _____

Quality:

① ② ③ ④ ⑤
⑥ ⑦ ⑧ ⑨ ⑩

RATE YOUR DAY
On track with goals?

| 10% | 20% | 30% | 40% | 50% | 60% | 70% | 80% | 90% | 100% |

DAY 2

Day of the Week/Date _____

TODAY'S FOCUS

☐ Arms ☐ Legs ☐ Core ☐ Chest ☐ Back ☐ Balance ☐ Flexibility ☐ Total-Body Conditioning

CARDIO

ACTIVITY	MINUTES	LEVEL/SPEED/ INTENSITY	HEART RATE	CALORIES BURNED	NOTES

STRENGTH

EXERCISE	SET 1		SET 2		SET 3		SET 4		SET 5	
	REPS	WEIGHT	REPS	WEIGHT	REPS	WEIGHT	REPS	WEIGHT	REPS	WEIGHT

STRETCHING/MOBILITY

ACTIVITY/MOVE	REPS/TIME	NOTES

WATCH YOUR BALANCE. *To avoid injury and muscle imbalances, aim for all-around training. Worked your squads hard? Give your hamstrings some attention, too. Pressing with your chest? Equal it out with some back work.*

NUTRITION

		TIME	CALORIES	PROTEIN	CARBS	FAT
BREAKFAST						
SNACK						
LUNCH						
SNACK						
DINNER						
SNACK						
DAILY TOTALS						

WATER (8-OZ SERVINGS)

○ ○ ○ ○ ○ ○ ○ ○ ○ ○ ○ ○ ○ ○ ○ ○

SUPPLEMENT	AMOUNT
_____	_____
_____	_____
_____	_____
_____	_____
_____	_____

SLEEP

Lights Out _____

Wake Up _____

Quality:

① ② ③ ④ ⑤
⑥ ⑦ ⑧ ⑨ ⑩

RATE YOUR DAY

On track with goals?

| 10% | 20% | 30% | 40% | 50% | 60% | 70% | 80% | 90% | 100% |

TRACK IT

DAY 3

Day of the Week/Date _____

TODAY'S FOCUS

☐ Arms ☐ Legs ☐ Core ☐ Chest ☐ Back ☐ Balance ☐ Flexibility ☐ Total-Body Conditioning

CARDIO

ACTIVITY	MINUTES	LEVEL/SPEED/INTENSITY	HEART RATE	CALORIES BURNED	NOTES

STRENGTH

EXERCISE	SET 1		SET 2		SET 3		SET 4		SET 5	
	REPS	WEIGHT	REPS	WEIGHT	REPS	WEIGHT	REPS	WEIGHT	REPS	WEIGHT

STRETCHING/MOBILITY

ACTIVITY/MOVE	REPS/TIME	NOTES

CRUSH THE BARRIERS.

"There are no limits. There are plateaus, but you must not stay there, you must go beyond them." —Bruce Lee

NUTRITION

	TIME	CALORIES	PROTEIN	CARBS	FAT
BREAKFAST					
SNACK					
LUNCH					
SNACK					
DINNER					
SNACK					
DAILY TOTALS					

WATER (8-OZ SERVINGS)

○ ○ ○ ○ ○ ○ ○ ○ ○ ○ ○ ○ ○ ○ ○

SUPPLEMENT	AMOUNT
_____	_____
_____	_____
_____	_____
_____	_____
_____	_____

SLEEP

Lights Out _____

Wake Up _____

Quality:

① ② ③ ④ ⑤
⑥ ⑦ ⑧ ⑨ ⑩

RATE YOUR DAY

On track with goals?

10%　20%　30%　40%　50%　60%　70%　80%　90%　100%

DAY 4

Day of the Week/Date _____

TODAY'S FOCUS

☐ Arms ☐ Legs ☐ Core ☐ Chest ☐ Back ☐ Balance ☐ Flexibility ☐ Total-Body Conditioning

CARDIO

ACTIVITY	MINUTES	LEVEL/SPEED/INTENSITY	HEART RATE	CALORIES BURNED	NOTES

STRENGTH

EXERCISE	SET 1		SET 2		SET 3		SET 4		SET 5	
	REPS	WEIGHT	REPS	WEIGHT	REPS	WEIGHT	REPS	WEIGHT	REPS	WEIGHT

STRETCHING/MOBILITY

ACTIVITY/MOVE	REPS/TIME	NOTES

BUST THIS EXCUSE. *The top reason people skip workouts? Not feeling confident, according to a survey of 1,000. Man up and get some tips from your gym's trainers, a trusted fitness mag, or your most-ripped friend.*

NUTRITION

	TIME	CALORIES	PROTEIN	CARBS	FAT
BREAKFAST					
SNACK					
LUNCH					
SNACK					
DINNER					
SNACK					
DAILY TOTALS					

WATER (8-OZ SERVINGS)

○ ○ ○ ○ ○ ○ ○ ○ ○ ○ ○ ○ ○ ○ ○

SUPPLEMENT   **AMOUNT**

_____ | _____
_____ | _____
_____ | _____
_____ | _____
_____ | _____

SLEEP

Lights Out _____

Wake Up _____

Quality:

① ② ③ ④ ⑤
⑥ ⑦ ⑧ ⑨ ⑩

RATE YOUR DAY

On track with goals?

| 10% | 20% | 30% | 40% | 50% | 60% | 70% | 80% | 90% | 100% |

TRACK IT

DAY 5

Day of the Week/Date _____

TODAY'S FOCUS

☐ Arms ☐ Legs ☐ Core ☐ Chest ☐ Back ☐ Balance ☐ Flexibility ☐ Total-Body Conditioning

CARDIO

ACTIVITY	MINUTES	LEVEL/SPEED/ INTENSITY	HEART RATE	CALORIES BURNED	NOTES

STRENGTH

EXERCISE	SET 1		SET 2		SET 3		SET 4		SET 5	
	REPS	WEIGHT	REPS	WEIGHT	REPS	WEIGHT	REPS	WEIGHT	REPS	WEIGHT

STRETCHING/MOBILITY

ACTIVITY/MOVE	REPS/TIME	NOTES

DRINK BEET JUICE. *Researchers found that beet juice may reduce muscle soreness from intense exercise. In another study, soccer players who drank concentrated beet juice ran farther while keeping their heart rates stable.*

NUTRITION

		TIME	CALORIES	PROTEIN	CARBS	FAT
BREAKFAST						
SNACK						
LUNCH						
SNACK						
DINNER						
SNACK						
DAILY TOTALS						

WATER (8-OZ SERVINGS)

○ ○ ○ ○ ○ ○ ○ ○ ○ ○ ○ ○ ○ ○ ○

SUPPLEMENT	**AMOUNT**
_____	_____
_____	_____
_____	_____
_____	_____
_____	_____

SLEEP

Lights Out _____

Wake Up _____

Quality:

① ② ③ ④ ⑤
⑥ ⑦ ⑧ ⑨ ⑩

RATE YOUR DAY
On track with goals?

| 10% | 20% | 30% | 40% | 50% | 60% | 70% | 80% | 90% | 100% |

TRACK IT

DAY 6

Day of the Week/Date _____

TODAY'S FOCUS

☐ Arms ☐ Legs ☐ Core ☐ Chest ☐ Back ☐ Balance ☐ Flexibility ☐ Total-Body Conditioning

CARDIO

ACTIVITY	MINUTES	LEVEL/SPEED/INTENSITY	HEART RATE	CALORIES BURNED	NOTES

STRENGTH

EXERCISE	SET 1		SET 2		SET 3		SET 4		SET 5	
	REPS	WEIGHT	REPS	WEIGHT	REPS	WEIGHT	REPS	WEIGHT	REPS	WEIGHT

STRETCHING/MOBILITY

ACTIVITY/MOVE	REPS/TIME	NOTES

HOW ARE YOUR STEPS?

"When it is obvious that the goals cannot be reached, don't adjust the goals; adjust the action steps." —Confucius

NUTRITION

		TIME	CALORIES	PROTEIN	CARBS	FAT
BREAKFAST						
SNACK						
LUNCH						
SNACK						
DINNER						
SNACK						
DAILY TOTALS						

WATER (8-OZ SERVINGS)

○ ○ ○ ○ ○ ○ ○ ○ ○ ○ ○ ○ ○ ○ ○

SUPPLEMENT	AMOUNT	SLEEP
_____	_____	Lights Out _____
_____	_____	Wake Up _____
_____	_____	Quality:
_____	_____	① ② ③ ④ ⑤
_____	_____	⑥ ⑦ ⑧ ⑨ ⑩

RATE YOUR DAY
On track with goals?

10%	20%	30%	40%	50%	60%	70%	80%	90%	100%

TRACK IT

DAY 7

Day of the Week/Date _____

TODAY'S FOCUS

☐ Arms ☐ Legs ☐ Core ☐ Chest ☐ Back ☐ Balance ☐ Flexibility ☐ Total-Body Conditioning

CARDIO

ACTIVITY	MINUTES	LEVEL/SPEED/INTENSITY	HEART RATE	CALORIES BURNED	NOTES

STRENGTH

EXERCISE	SET 1		SET 2		SET 3		SET 4		SET 5	
	REPS	WEIGHT	REPS	WEIGHT	REPS	WEIGHT	REPS	WEIGHT	REPS	WEIGHT

STRETCHING/MOBILITY

ACTIVITY/MOVE	REPS/TIME	NOTES

CELEBRATE WEEK 8! *Record your gains on pages 10 and 11. But also look for gaps or weaknesses. Is anything holding you back from your goals that you need to focus on?*

NUTRITION

		TIME	CALORIES	PROTEIN	CARBS	FAT
BREAKFAST						
SNACK						
LUNCH						
SNACK						
DINNER						
SNACK						
DAILY TOTALS						

WATER (8-OZ SERVINGS)

○ ○ ○ ○ ○ ○ ○ ○ ○ ○ ○ ○ ○ ○ ○

SUPPLEMENT   AMOUNT

_____ | _____
_____ | _____
_____ | _____
_____ | _____
_____ | _____

SLEEP

Lights Out _____

Wake Up _____

Quality:

① ② ③ ④ ⑤
⑥ ⑦ ⑧ ⑨ ⑩

RATE YOUR DAY
On track with goals?

| 10% | 20% | 30% | 40% | 50% | 60% | 70% | 80% | 90% | 100% |

MAP IT

FITNESS

	CARDIO	STRENGTH	STRETCHING/ MOBILITY
DAY 1			
DAY 2			
DAY 3			
DAY 4			
DAY 5			
DAY 6			
DAY 7			

NOTES

_____

_____

_____

_____

NUTRITION

	BREAKFAST	LUNCH	DINNER	SNACKS
DAY 1				
DAY 2				
DAY 3				
DAY 4				
DAY 5				
DAY 6				
DAY 7				

NOTES

_____
_____
_____
_____

TRACK IT

DAY 1

Day of the Week/Date _____

TODAY'S FOCUS

☐ Arms ☐ Legs ☐ Core ☐ Chest ☐ Back ☐ Balance ☐ Flexibility ☐ Total-Body Conditioning

CARDIO

ACTIVITY	MINUTES	LEVEL/SPEED/INTENSITY	HEART RATE	CALORIES BURNED	NOTES

STRENGTH

EXERCISE	SET 1		SET 2		SET 3		SET 4		SET 5	
	REPS	WEIGHT	REPS	WEIGHT	REPS	WEIGHT	REPS	WEIGHT	REPS	WEIGHT

STRETCHING/MOBILITY

ACTIVITY/MOVE	REPS/TIME	NOTES

ALL ATTENTION TO YOUR ABS. *Reverse crunches are a great move toward a six-pack—if you don't cheat the effort. Before raising your legs, round your back by rolling your hips and pelvis toward your chest.*

NUTRITION

		TIME	CALORIES	PROTEIN	CARBS	FAT
BREAKFAST						
SNACK						
LUNCH						
SNACK						
DINNER						
SNACK						
DAILY TOTALS						

WATER (8-OZ SERVINGS)

○ ○ ○ ○ ○ ○ ○ ○ ○ ○ ○ ○ ○ ○ ○ ○

SUPPLEMENT   **AMOUNT**

_____ | _____
_____ | _____
_____ | _____
_____ | _____
_____ | _____

SLEEP

Lights Out _____

Wake Up _____

Quality:

① ② ③ ④ ⑤
⑥ ⑦ ⑧ ⑨ ⑩

RATE YOUR DAY
On track with goals?

| 10% | 20% | 30% | 40% | 50% | 60% | 70% | 80% | 90% | 100% |

TRACK IT

DAY 2

Day of the Week/Date _____

TODAY'S FOCUS

☐ Arms ☐ Legs ☐ Core ☐ Chest ☐ Back ☐ Balance ☐ Flexibility ☐ Total-Body Conditioning

CARDIO

ACTIVITY	MINUTES	LEVEL/SPEED/INTENSITY	HEART RATE	CALORIES BURNED	NOTES

STRENGTH

EXERCISE	SET 1		SET 2		SET 3		SET 4		SET 5	
	REPS	WEIGHT	REPS	WEIGHT	REPS	WEIGHT	REPS	WEIGHT	REPS	WEIGHT

STRETCHING/MOBILITY

ACTIVITY/MOVE	REPS/TIME	NOTES

PROGRESS ON THE FLOOR. *The classic push-up is a great indicator of upper-body strength, specifically in your chest, triceps, and core. Try to push the number you can do (with good form!) over the next few weeks.*

NUTRITION

		TIME	CALORIES	PROTEIN	CARBS	FAT
BREAKFAST						
SNACK						
LUNCH						
SNACK						
DINNER						
SNACK						
DAILY TOTALS						

WATER (8-OZ SERVINGS)

○ ○ ○ ○ ○ ○ ○ ○ ○ ○ ○ ○ ○ ○ ○ ○

SUPPLEMENT	AMOUNT
_____	_____
_____	_____
_____	_____
_____	_____
_____	_____

SLEEP

Lights Out _____

Wake Up _____

Quality:

① ② ③ ④ ⑤
⑥ ⑦ ⑧ ⑨ ⑩

RATE YOUR DAY
On track with goals?

| 10% | 20% | 30% | 40% | 50% | 60% | 70% | 80% | 90% | 100% |

DAY 3

Day of the Week/Date _____

TODAY'S FOCUS

☐ Arms ☐ Legs ☐ Core ☐ Chest ☐ Back ☐ Balance ☐ Flexibility ☐ Total-Body Conditioning

CARDIO

ACTIVITY	MINUTES	LEVEL/SPEED/INTENSITY	HEART RATE	CALORIES BURNED	NOTES

STRENGTH

EXERCISE	SET 1		SET 2		SET 3		SET 4		SET 5	
	REPS	WEIGHT	REPS	WEIGHT	REPS	WEIGHT	REPS	WEIGHT	REPS	WEIGHT

STRETCHING/MOBILITY

ACTIVITY/MOVE	REPS/TIME	NOTES

KEEP CHALLENGING YOURSELF.

"Good is not good when better is expected." —*Vin Scully*

NUTRITION

		TIME	CALORIES	PROTEIN	CARBS	FAT
BREAKFAST						
SNACK						
LUNCH						
SNACK						
DINNER						
SNACK						
DAILY TOTALS						

WATER (8-OZ SERVINGS)

○ ○ ○ ○ ○ ○ ○ ○ ○ ○ ○ ○ ○ ○ ○

SUPPLEMENT	AMOUNT
_____	_____
_____	_____
_____	_____
_____	_____
_____	_____

SLEEP

Lights Out _____

Wake Up _____

Quality:

① ② ③ ④ ⑤
⑥ ⑦ ⑧ ⑨ ⑩

RATE YOUR DAY

On track with goals?

10%　20%　30%　40%　50%　60%　70%　80%　90%　100%

TRACK IT

DAY 4

Day of the Week/Date _____

TODAY'S FOCUS

☐ Arms ☐ Legs ☐ Core ☐ Chest ☐ Back ☐ Balance ☐ Flexibility ☐ Total-Body Conditioning

CARDIO

ACTIVITY	MINUTES	LEVEL/SPEED/INTENSITY	HEART RATE	CALORIES BURNED	NOTES

STRENGTH

EXERCISE	SET 1		SET 2		SET 3		SET 4		SET 5	
	REPS	WEIGHT	REPS	WEIGHT	REPS	WEIGHT	REPS	WEIGHT	REPS	WEIGHT

STRETCHING/MOBILITY

ACTIVITY/MOVE	REPS/TIME	NOTES

SEE IT. *Having trouble pushing out that last rep or completing that last mile? See yourself doing it. Visualization may sound hokey, but many sports psychologists swear by it. Try it and see if it works for you.*

NUTRITION

		TIME	CALORIES	PROTEIN	CARBS	FAT
BREAKFAST						
SNACK						
LUNCH						
SNACK						
DINNER						
SNACK						
DAILY TOTALS						

WATER (8-OZ SERVINGS)

○ ○ ○ ○ ○ ○ ○ ○ ○ ○ ○ ○ ○ ○ ○ ○

SUPPLEMENT	**AMOUNT**
_____	_____
_____	_____
_____	_____
_____	_____
_____	_____

SLEEP

Lights Out _____

Wake Up _____

Quality:

① ② ③ ④ ⑤
⑥ ⑦ ⑧ ⑨ ⑩

RATE YOUR DAY

On track with goals?

| 10% | 20% | 30% | 40% | 50% | 60% | 70% | 80% | 90% | 100% |

TRACK IT

DAY 5

Day of the Week/Date _____

TODAY'S FOCUS

☐ Arms ☐ Legs ☐ Core ☐ Chest ☐ Back ☐ Balance ☐ Flexibility ☐ Total-Body Conditioning

CARDIO

ACTIVITY	MINUTES	LEVEL/SPEED/INTENSITY	HEART RATE	CALORIES BURNED	NOTES

STRENGTH

EXERCISE	SET 1		SET 2		SET 3		SET 4		SET 5	
	REPS	WEIGHT	REPS	WEIGHT	REPS	WEIGHT	REPS	WEIGHT	REPS	WEIGHT

STRETCHING/MOBILITY

ACTIVITY/MOVE	REPS/TIME	NOTES

WALK TO THE FINISH LINE LIKE A FARMER. *Farmer's walks build strength and a stable core. If you save them until the end of your workout, they help you sneak in a little more weight work when your energy is waning.*

NUTRITION

		TIME	CALORIES	PROTEIN	CARBS	FAT
BREAKFAST						
SNACK						
LUNCH						
SNACK						
DINNER						
SNACK						
DAILY TOTALS						

WATER (8-OZ SERVINGS)

○ ○ ○ ○ ○ ○ ○ ○ ○ ○ ○ ○ ○ ○ ○

SUPPLEMENT	AMOUNT
_____	_____
_____	_____
_____	_____
_____	_____
_____	_____

SLEEP

Lights Out _____

Wake Up _____

Quality:

① ② ③ ④ ⑤
⑥ ⑦ ⑧ ⑨ ⑩

RATE YOUR DAY

On track with goals?

10%   20%   30%   40%   50%   60%   70%   80%   90%   100%

DAY 6

Day of the Week/Date _____

TODAY'S FOCUS

☐ Arms ☐ Legs ☐ Core ☐ Chest ☐ Back ☐ Balance ☐ Flexibility ☐ Total-Body Conditioning

CARDIO

ACTIVITY	MINUTES	LEVEL/SPEED/INTENSITY	HEART RATE	CALORIES BURNED	NOTES

STRENGTH

EXERCISE	SET 1		SET 2		SET 3		SET 4		SET 5	
	REPS	WEIGHT	REPS	WEIGHT	REPS	WEIGHT	REPS	WEIGHT	REPS	WEIGHT

STRETCHING/MOBILITY

ACTIVITY/MOVE	REPS/TIME	NOTES

STAY FOCUSED ON YOUR GOALS.

"Today I will do what others won't, so tomorrow I can accomplish what others can't." —Jerry Rice

NUTRITION

		TIME	CALORIES	PROTEIN	CARBS	FAT
BREAKFAST						
SNACK						
LUNCH						
SNACK						
DINNER						
SNACK						
DAILY TOTALS						

WATER (8-OZ SERVINGS)

○ ○ ○ ○ ○ ○ ○ ○ ○ ○ ○ ○ ○ ○ ○

SUPPLEMENT	AMOUNT
_____	_____
_____	_____
_____	_____
_____	_____
_____	_____

SLEEP

Lights Out _____

Wake Up _____

Quality:

① ② ③ ④ ⑤
⑥ ⑦ ⑧ ⑨ ⑩

RATE YOUR DAY

On track with goals?

| 10% | 20% | 30% | 40% | 50% | 60% | 70% | 80% | 90% | 100% |

— — TRACK IT — —

DAY 7

Day of the Week/Date _____

TODAY'S FOCUS

☐ Arms ☐ Legs ☐ Core ☐ Chest ☐ Back ☐ Balance ☐ Flexibility ☐ Total-Body Conditioning

CARDIO

ACTIVITY	MINUTES	LEVEL/SPEED/INTENSITY	HEART RATE	CALORIES BURNED	NOTES

STRENGTH

EXERCISE	SET 1		SET 2		SET 3		SET 4		SET 5	
	REPS	WEIGHT	REPS	WEIGHT	REPS	WEIGHT	REPS	WEIGHT	REPS	WEIGHT

STRETCHING/MOBILITY

ACTIVITY/MOVE	REPS/TIME	NOTES

RACK IT UP! *It's time to pen in your weekly progress on pages 10 and 11. Keep your workout journal in a spot where you can see it beyond the gym to stay focused on your goals and successes.*

NUTRITION

	TIME	CALORIES	PROTEIN	CARBS	FAT
BREAKFAST					
SNACK					
LUNCH					
SNACK					
DINNER					
SNACK					
DAILY TOTALS					

WATER (8-OZ SERVINGS)

○ ○ ○ ○ ○ ○ ○ ○ ○ ○ ○ ○ ○ ○ ○ ○

SUPPLEMENT	AMOUNT
_____	_____
_____	_____
_____	_____
_____	_____
_____	_____

SLEEP

Lights Out _____

Wake Up _____

Quality:

① ② ③ ④ ⑤

⑥ ⑦ ⑧ ⑨ ⑩

RATE YOUR DAY

On track with goals?

| 10% | 20% | 30% | 40% | 50% | 60% | 70% | 80% | 90% | 100% |

MAP IT

FITNESS

	CARDIO	STRENGTH	STRETCHING/ MOBILITY
DAY 1			
DAY 2			
DAY 3			
DAY 4			
DAY 5			
DAY 6			
DAY 7			

NOTES

_____
_____
_____
_____

NUTRITION

	BREAKFAST	LUNCH	DINNER	SNACKS
DAY 1				
DAY 2				
DAY 3				
DAY 4				
DAY 5				
DAY 6				
DAY 7				

NOTES

TRACK IT

DAY 1

Day of the Week/Date _____

TODAY'S FOCUS

☐ Arms ☐ Legs ☐ Core ☐ Chest ☐ Back ☐ Balance ☐ Flexibility ☐ Total-Body Conditioning

CARDIO

ACTIVITY	MINUTES	LEVEL/SPEED/INTENSITY	HEART RATE	CALORIES BURNED	NOTES

STRENGTH

EXERCISE	SET 1		SET 2		SET 3		SET 4		SET 5	
	REPS	WEIGHT	REPS	WEIGHT	REPS	WEIGHT	REPS	WEIGHT	REPS	WEIGHT

STRETCHING/MOBILITY

ACTIVITY/MOVE	REPS/TIME	NOTES

POWER TO THE PLANK. *Having a strong core protects you from injury and helps you lift more weight. Add the move to your workouts a few times a week, aiming for the maximum time you can hold with good form.*

NUTRITION

		TIME	CALORIES	PROTEIN	CARBS	FAT
BREAKFAST						
SNACK						
LUNCH						
SNACK						
DINNER						
SNACK						
	DAILY TOTALS					

WATER (8-OZ SERVINGS)

○ ○ ○ ○ ○ ○ ○ ○ ○ ○ ○ ○ ○ ○ ○ ○

SUPPLEMENT   **AMOUNT**

_____ : _____

_____ : _____

_____ : _____

_____ : _____

_____ : _____

SLEEP

Lights Out _____

Wake Up _____

Quality:

① ② ③ ④ ⑤

⑥ ⑦ ⑧ ⑨ ⑩

RATE YOUR DAY

On track with goals?

| 10% | 20% | 30% | 40% | 50% | 60% | 70% | 80% | 90% | 100% |

DAY 2

Day of the Week/Date _____

TODAY'S FOCUS

☐ Arms ☐ Legs ☐ Core ☐ Chest ☐ Back ☐ Balance ☐ Flexibility ☐ Total-Body Conditioning

CARDIO

ACTIVITY	MINUTES	LEVEL/SPEED/INTENSITY	HEART RATE	CALORIES BURNED	NOTES

STRENGTH

EXERCISE	SET 1		SET 2		SET 3		SET 4		SET 5	
	REPS	WEIGHT	REPS	WEIGHT	REPS	WEIGHT	REPS	WEIGHT	REPS	WEIGHT

STRETCHING/MOBILITY

ACTIVITY/MOVE	REPS/TIME	NOTES

DRINK IN NATURAL RECOVERY. *Tart cherry juice serves up anthocyanins, natural anti-inflammatory compounds that can reduce muscle soreness. Just make sure you choose unsweetened juice to get the most benefit.*

NUTRITION

		TIME	CALORIES	PROTEIN	CARBS	FAT
BREAKFAST						
SNACK						
LUNCH						
SNACK						
DINNER						
SNACK						
	DAILY TOTALS					

WATER (8-OZ SERVINGS)

○ ○ ○ ○ ○ ○ ○ ○ ○ ○ ○ ○ ○ ○ ○

SUPPLEMENT   **AMOUNT**

_____ | _____

_____ | _____

_____ | _____

_____ | _____

_____ | _____

SLEEP

Lights Out _____

Wake Up _____

Quality:

① ② ③ ④ ⑤

⑥ ⑦ ⑧ ⑨ ⑩

RATE YOUR DAY
On track with goals?

| 10% | 20% | 30% | 40% | 50% | 60% | 70% | 80% | 90% | 100% |

TRACK IT

DAY 3

Day of the Week/Date _____

TODAY'S FOCUS

☐ Arms ☐ Legs ☐ Core ☐ Chest ☐ Back ☐ Balance ☐ Flexibility ☐ Total-Body Conditioning

CARDIO

ACTIVITY	MINUTES	LEVEL/SPEED/INTENSITY	HEART RATE	CALORIES BURNED	NOTES

STRENGTH

EXERCISE	SET 1		SET 2		SET 3		SET 4		SET 5	
	REPS	WEIGHT	REPS	WEIGHT	REPS	WEIGHT	REPS	WEIGHT	REPS	WEIGHT

STRETCHING/MOBILITY

ACTIVITY/MOVE	REPS/TIME	NOTES

KEEP GETTING STRONGER.

"The principle is competing against yourself. It's about self-improvement, about being better than you were the day before." —*Steve Young*

NUTRITION

	TIME	CALORIES	PROTEIN	CARBS	FAT
BREAKFAST					
SNACK					
LUNCH					
SNACK					
DINNER					
SNACK					
DAILY TOTALS					

WATER (8-OZ SERVINGS)

○ ○ ○ ○ ○ ○ ○ ○ ○ ○ ○ ○ ○ ○

SUPPLEMENT   **AMOUNT**

_____ | _____
_____ | _____
_____ | _____
_____ | _____
_____ | _____

SLEEP

Lights Out _____

Wake Up _____

Quality:

① ② ③ ④ ⑤
⑥ ⑦ ⑧ ⑨ ⑩

RATE YOUR DAY

On track with goals?

| 10% | 20% | 30% | 40% | 50% | 60% | 70% | 80% | 90% | 100% |

TRACK IT

DAY 4

Day of the Week/Date _____

TODAY'S FOCUS

☐ Arms ☐ Legs ☐ Core ☐ Chest ☐ Back ☐ Balance ☐ Flexibility ☐ Total-Body Conditioning

CARDIO

ACTIVITY	MINUTES	LEVEL/SPEED/INTENSITY	HEART RATE	CALORIES BURNED	NOTES

STRENGTH

EXERCISE	SET 1		SET 2		SET 3		SET 4		SET 5	
	REPS	WEIGHT	REPS	WEIGHT	REPS	WEIGHT	REPS	WEIGHT	REPS	WEIGHT

STRETCHING/MOBILITY

ACTIVITY/MOVE	REPS/TIME	NOTES

GO TO THE ROPES. *Battle ropes can help you burn fat and build muscle at the same time. Rope slams and circles are popular moves to try, but ask a trainer for ways to use ropes to meet your specific goals.*

NUTRITION

		TIME	CALORIES	PROTEIN	CARBS	FAT
BREAKFAST						
SNACK						
LUNCH						
SNACK						
DINNER						
SNACK						
DAILY TOTALS						

WATER (8-OZ SERVINGS)

○ ○ ○ ○ ○ ○ ○ ○ ○ ○ ○ ○ ○ ○

SUPPLEMENT	AMOUNT
_____	_____
_____	_____
_____	_____
_____	_____
_____	_____

SLEEP

Lights Out _____

Wake Up _____

Quality:

① ② ③ ④ ⑤
⑥ ⑦ ⑧ ⑨ ⑩

RATE YOUR DAY
On track with goals?

| 10% | 20% | 30% | 40% | 50% | 60% | 70% | 80% | 90% | 100% |

DAY 5

Day of the Week/Date _____

TODAY'S FOCUS

☐ Arms ☐ Legs ☐ Core ☐ Chest ☐ Back ☐ Balance ☐ Flexibility ☐ Total-Body Conditioning

CARDIO

ACTIVITY	MINUTES	LEVEL/SPEED/INTENSITY	HEART RATE	CALORIES BURNED	NOTES

STRENGTH

EXERCISE	SET 1		SET 2		SET 3		SET 4		SET 5	
	REPS	WEIGHT	REPS	WEIGHT	REPS	WEIGHT	REPS	WEIGHT	REPS	WEIGHT

STRETCHING/MOBILITY

ACTIVITY/MOVE	REPS/TIME	NOTES

THINK DOWN, NOT UP. *To make pull-ups feel easier and crank out more reps, think about pulling your elbows down and back as if they were reaching for your back pockets. So simple but it works!*

NUTRITION

		TIME	CALORIES	PROTEIN	CARBS	FAT
BREAKFAST						
SNACK						
LUNCH						
SNACK						
DINNER						
SNACK						
	DAILY TOTALS					

WATER (8-OZ SERVINGS)

○ ○ ○ ○ ○ ○ ○ ○ ○ ○ ○ ○ ○ ○ ○

SUPPLEMENT   **AMOUNT**

_____ | _____

_____ | _____

_____ | _____

_____ | _____

_____ | _____

SLEEP

Lights Out _____

Wake Up _____

Quality:

① ② ③ ④ ⑤
⑥ ⑦ ⑧ ⑨ ⑩

RATE YOUR DAY
On track with goals?

| 10% | 20% | 30% | 40% | 50% | 60% | 70% | 80% | 90% | 100% |

DAY 6

Day of the Week/Date _____

TODAY'S FOCUS

☐ Arms ☐ Legs ☐ Core ☐ Chest ☐ Back ☐ Balance ☐ Flexibility ☐ Total-Body Conditioning

CARDIO

ACTIVITY	MINUTES	LEVEL/SPEED/INTENSITY	HEART RATE	CALORIES BURNED	NOTES

STRENGTH

EXERCISE	SET 1		SET 2		SET 3		SET 4		SET 5	
	REPS	WEIGHT	REPS	WEIGHT	REPS	WEIGHT	REPS	WEIGHT	REPS	WEIGHT

STRETCHING/MOBILITY

ACTIVITY/MOVE	REPS/TIME	NOTES

WHEN YOU HAVE A ROUGH WEEK, QUICKLY REGROUP.

"Losers live in the past. Winners learn from the past and enjoy working in the present toward the future." —Denis Waitley

NUTRITION

		TIME	CALORIES	PROTEIN	CARBS	FAT
BREAKFAST						
SNACK						
LUNCH						
SNACK						
DINNER						
SNACK						
DAILY TOTALS						

WATER (8-OZ SERVINGS)

○ ○ ○ ○ ○ ○ ○ ○ ○ ○ ○ ○ ○ ○ ○

SUPPLEMENT	AMOUNT
_____	_____
_____	_____
_____	_____
_____	_____
_____	_____

SLEEP

Lights Out _____

Wake Up _____

Quality:

① ② ③ ④ ⑤
⑥ ⑦ ⑧ ⑨ ⑩

RATE YOUR DAY
On track with goals?

| 10% | 20% | 30% | 40% | 50% | 60% | 70% | 80% | 90% | 100% |

TRACK IT — —

DAY 7

Day of the Week/Date _____

TODAY'S FOCUS

☐ Arms ☐ Legs ☐ Core ☐ Chest ☐ Back ☐ Balance ☐ Flexibility ☐ Total-Body Conditioning

CARDIO

ACTIVITY	MINUTES	LEVEL/SPEED/ INTENSITY	HEART RATE	CALORIES BURNED	NOTES

STRENGTH

EXERCISE	SET 1		SET 2		SET 3		SET 4		SET 5	
	REPS	WEIGHT	REPS	WEIGHT	REPS	WEIGHT	REPS	WEIGHT	REPS	WEIGHT

STRETCHING/MOBILITY

ACTIVITY/MOVE	REPS/TIME	NOTES

KNOW THE NUMBERS. *Track this week's progress on pages 10 and 11. Choose the number you're most proud of to post on a sticky note and put in a prominent place—your bathroom mirror or your dashboard.*

NUTRITION

		TIME	CALORIES	PROTEIN	CARBS	FAT
BREAKFAST						
SNACK						
LUNCH						
SNACK						
DINNER						
SNACK						
DAILY TOTALS						

WATER (8-OZ SERVINGS)

○ ○ ○ ○ ○ ○ ○ ○ ○ ○ ○ ○ ○ ○ ○ ○

SUPPLEMENT	AMOUNT
_____	_____
_____	_____
_____	_____
_____	_____
_____	_____

SLEEP

Lights Out _____

Wake Up _____

Quality:

① ② ③ ④ ⑤
⑥ ⑦ ⑧ ⑨ ⑩

RATE YOUR DAY
On track with goals?

| 10% | 20% | 30% | 40% | 50% | 60% | 70% | 80% | 90% | 100% |

MAP IT

FITNESS

	CARDIO	STRENGTH	STRETCHING/ MOBILITY
DAY 1			
DAY 2			
DAY 3			
DAY 4			
DAY 5			
DAY 6			
DAY 7			

NOTES

— — — — DATES:

NUTRITION

	BREAKFAST	LUNCH	DINNER	SNACKS
DAY 1				
DAY 2				
DAY 3				
DAY 4				
DAY 5				
DAY 6				
DAY 7				

NOTES

_____

_____

_____

_____

TRACK IT

DAY 1

Day of the Week/Date _____

TODAY'S FOCUS

☐ Arms ☐ Legs ☐ Core ☐ Chest ☐ Back ☐ Balance ☐ Flexibility ☐ Total-Body Conditioning

CARDIO

ACTIVITY	MINUTES	LEVEL/SPEED/INTENSITY	HEART RATE	CALORIES BURNED	NOTES

STRENGTH

EXERCISE	SET 1		SET 2		SET 3		SET 4		SET 5	
	REPS	WEIGHT	REPS	WEIGHT	REPS	WEIGHT	REPS	WEIGHT	REPS	WEIGHT

STRETCHING/MOBILITY

ACTIVITY/MOVE	REPS/TIME	NOTES

SOAK IN SALT. *Add ¼ cup of Epsom salts to your bathwater to boost your body's store of magnesium—it's absorbed by the skin. The mineral is great for fighting aches and pains, particularly after strenuous exercise.*

NUTRITION

		TIME	CALORIES	PROTEIN	CARBS	FAT
BREAKFAST						
SNACK						
LUNCH						
SNACK						
DINNER						
SNACK						
DAILY TOTALS						

WATER (8-OZ SERVINGS)

○ ○ ○ ○ ○ ○ ○ ○ ○ ○ ○ ○ ○ ○ ○ ○

SUPPLEMENT	AMOUNT
_____	_____
_____	_____
_____	_____
_____	_____
_____	_____

SLEEP

Lights Out _____

Wake Up _____

Quality:

① ② ③ ④ ⑤
⑥ ⑦ ⑧ ⑨ ⑩

RATE YOUR DAY
On track with goals?

| 10% | 20% | 30% | 40% | 50% | 60% | 70% | 80% | 90% | 100% |

DAY 2
Day of the Week/Date _____

TODAY'S FOCUS
☐ Arms ☐ Legs ☐ Core ☐ Chest ☐ Back ☐ Balance ☐ Flexibility ☐ Total-Body Conditioning

CARDIO

ACTIVITY	MINUTES	LEVEL/SPEED/ INTENSITY	HEART RATE	CALORIES BURNED	NOTES

STRENGTH

EXERCISE	SET 1		SET 2		SET 3		SET 4		SET 5	
	REPS	WEIGHT	REPS	WEIGHT	REPS	WEIGHT	REPS	WEIGHT	REPS	WEIGHT

STRETCHING/MOBILITY

ACTIVITY/MOVE	REPS/TIME	NOTES

STAY WELL FOR WORKOUTS. *Keep your immune system revved with probiotic-rich foods and drinks, such as kimchi, kombucha, kefir, miso, pickles, sauerkraut, tempeh, and unsweetened Greek yogurt.*

NUTRITION

		TIME	CALORIES	PROTEIN	CARBS	FAT
BREAKFAST						
SNACK						
LUNCH						
SNACK						
DINNER						
SNACK						
DAILY TOTALS						

WATER (8-OZ SERVINGS)

○ ○ ○ ○ ○ ○ ○ ○ ○ ○ ○ ○ ○ ○

SUPPLEMENT | **AMOUNT**

_____ | _____
_____ | _____
_____ | _____
_____ | _____
_____ | _____

SLEEP

Lights Out _____

Wake Up _____

Quality:

(1) (2) (3) (4) (5)
(6) (7) (8) (9) (10)

RATE YOUR DAY
On track with goals?

| 10% | 20% | 30% | 40% | 50% | 60% | 70% | 80% | 90% | 100% |

DAY 3

Day of the Week/Date _____

TODAY'S FOCUS

☐ Arms   ☐ Legs   ☐ Core   ☐ Chest   ☐ Back   ☐ Balance   ☐ Flexibility   ☐ Total-Body Conditioning

CARDIO

ACTIVITY	MINUTES	LEVEL/SPEED/INTENSITY	HEART RATE	CALORIES BURNED	NOTES

STRENGTH

EXERCISE	SET 1		SET 2		SET 3		SET 4		SET 5	
	REPS	WEIGHT	REPS	WEIGHT	REPS	WEIGHT	REPS	WEIGHT	REPS	WEIGHT

STRETCHING/MOBILITY

ACTIVITY/MOVE	REPS/TIME	NOTES

PUT IN YOUR MAX.

"Nobody who ever gave his best regretted it." —*George Halas*

NUTRITION

		TIME	CALORIES	PROTEIN	CARBS	FAT
BREAKFAST						
SNACK						
LUNCH						
SNACK						
DINNER						
SNACK						
DAILY TOTALS						

WATER (8-OZ SERVINGS)

○ ○ ○ ○ ○ ○ ○ ○ ○ ○ ○ ○ ○ ○

SUPPLEMENT	AMOUNT
_____	_____
_____	_____
_____	_____
_____	_____
_____	_____

SLEEP

Lights Out _____

Wake Up _____

Quality:

① ② ③ ④ ⑤
⑥ ⑦ ⑧ ⑨ ⑩

RATE YOUR DAY

On track with goals?

| 10% | 20% | 30% | 40% | 50% | 60% | 70% | 80% | 90% | 100% |

DAY 4

Day of the Week/Date _____

TODAY'S FOCUS

☐ Arms ☐ Legs ☐ Core ☐ Chest ☐ Back ☐ Balance ☐ Flexibility ☐ Total-Body Conditioning

CARDIO

ACTIVITY	MINUTES	LEVEL/SPEED/INTENSITY	HEART RATE	CALORIES BURNED	NOTES

STRENGTH

EXERCISE	SET 1		SET 2		SET 3		SET 4		SET 5	
	REPS	WEIGHT	REPS	WEIGHT	REPS	WEIGHT	REPS	WEIGHT	REPS	WEIGHT

STRETCHING/MOBILITY

ACTIVITY/MOVE	REPS/TIME	NOTES

WHAT'S YOUR TEMPO? *Your lifting and lowering speed can change how you work your muscles. Try shaking it up every once in a while—it will force your muscles to adapt to different stresses and strengthen in the process.*

NUTRITION

		TIME	CALORIES	PROTEIN	CARBS	FAT
BREAKFAST						
SNACK						
LUNCH						
SNACK						
DINNER						
SNACK						
DAILY TOTALS						

WATER (8-OZ SERVINGS)

○ ○ ○ ○ ○ ○ ○ ○ ○ ○ ○ ○ ○ ○ ○

SUPPLEMENT	AMOUNT
_____	_____
_____	_____
_____	_____
_____	_____
_____	_____

SLEEP

Lights Out _____

Wake Up _____

Quality:

① ② ③ ④ ⑤
⑥ ⑦ ⑧ ⑨ ⑩

RATE YOUR DAY

On track with goals?

| 10% | 20% | 30% | 40% | 50% | 60% | 70% | 80% | 90% | 100% |

TRACK IT

DAY 5

Day of the Week/Date _____

TODAY'S FOCUS

☐ Arms ☐ Legs ☐ Core ☐ Chest ☐ Back ☐ Balance ☐ Flexibility ☐ Total-Body Conditioning

CARDIO

ACTIVITY	MINUTES	LEVEL/SPEED/INTENSITY	HEART RATE	CALORIES BURNED	NOTES

STRENGTH

EXERCISE	SET 1		SET 2		SET 3		SET 4		SET 5	
	REPS	WEIGHT	REPS	WEIGHT	REPS	WEIGHT	REPS	WEIGHT	REPS	WEIGHT

STRETCHING/MOBILITY

ACTIVITY/MOVE	REPS/TIME	NOTES

NEED MOTIVATION? *Dedicate your workout to someone you'd like to lend symbolic strength—a family member who's ill or a friend going through a tough time. Write the name on a rubber band and wear it around your wrist.*

NUTRITION

		TIME	CALORIES	PROTEIN	CARBS	FAT
BREAKFAST						
SNACK						
LUNCH						
SNACK						
DINNER						
SNACK						
	DAILY TOTALS					

WATER (8-OZ SERVINGS)

○ ○ ○ ○ ○ ○ ○ ○ ○ ○ ○ ○ ○ ○ ○

SUPPLEMENT   **AMOUNT**

_____ _____

_____ _____

_____ _____

_____ _____

_____ _____

SLEEP

Lights Out _____

Wake Up _____

Quality:

① ② ③ ④ ⑤
⑥ ⑦ ⑧ ⑨ ⑩

RATE YOUR DAY

On track with goals?

| 10% | 20% | 30% | 40% | 50% | 60% | 70% | 80% | 90% | 100% |

TRACK IT

DAY 6

Day of the Week/Date _____

TODAY'S FOCUS

☐ Arms ☐ Legs ☐ Core ☐ Chest ☐ Back ☐ Balance ☐ Flexibility ☐ Total-Body Conditioning

CARDIO

ACTIVITY	MINUTES	LEVEL/SPEED/INTENSITY	HEART RATE	CALORIES BURNED	NOTES

STRENGTH

EXERCISE	SET 1		SET 2		SET 3		SET 4		SET 5	
	REPS	WEIGHT	REPS	WEIGHT	REPS	WEIGHT	REPS	WEIGHT	REPS	WEIGHT

STRETCHING/MOBILITY

ACTIVITY/MOVE	REPS/TIME	NOTES

DON'T STOP. *"The mind is the limit. As long as the mind can envision the fact that you can do something, you can do it, as long as you really believe 100 percent."* —Arnold Schwarzenegger

NUTRITION

		TIME	CALORIES	PROTEIN	CARBS	FAT
BREAKFAST						
SNACK						
LUNCH						
SNACK						
DINNER						
SNACK						
	DAILY TOTALS					

WATER (8-OZ SERVINGS)
○ ○ ○ ○ ○ ○ ○ ○ ○ ○ ○ ○ ○ ○ ○ ○

SUPPLEMENT	AMOUNT
_____	_____
_____	_____
_____	_____
_____	_____
_____	_____

SLEEP

Lights Out _____

Wake Up _____

Quality:

① ② ③ ④ ⑤
⑥ ⑦ ⑧ ⑨ ⑩

RATE YOUR DAY
On track with goals?

| 10% | 20% | 30% | 40% | 50% | 60% | 70% | 80% | 90% | 100% |

TRACK IT

DAY 7

Day of the Week/Date _____

TODAY'S FOCUS

☐ Arms ☐ Legs ☐ Core ☐ Chest ☐ Back ☐ Balance ☐ Flexibility ☐ Total-Body Conditioning

CARDIO

ACTIVITY	MINUTES	LEVEL/SPEED/ INTENSITY	HEART RATE	CALORIES BURNED	NOTES

STRENGTH

EXERCISE	SET 1		SET 2		SET 3		SET 4		SET 5	
	REPS	WEIGHT	REPS	WEIGHT	REPS	WEIGHT	REPS	WEIGHT	REPS	WEIGHT

STRETCHING/MOBILITY

ACTIVITY/MOVE	REPS/TIME	NOTES

WEEK 11 DOWN! *Track this week's progress on pages 10 and 11. With two weeks to go in this training cycle, are there specific numbers or goals that need extra focus? Plan weeks 12 and 13 with these factors in mind.*

NUTRITION

		TIME	CALORIES	PROTEIN	CARBS	FAT
BREAKFAST						
SNACK						
LUNCH						
SNACK						
DINNER						
SNACK						
DAILY TOTALS						

WATER (8-OZ SERVINGS)

○ ○ ○ ○ ○ ○ ○ ○ ○ ○ ○ ○ ○ ○ ○ ○

SUPPLEMENT	**AMOUNT**
_____	_____
_____	_____
_____	_____
_____	_____
_____	_____

SLEEP

Lights Out _____

Wake Up _____

Quality:

(1) (2) (3) (4) (5)
(6) (7) (8) (9) (10)

RATE YOUR DAY
On track with goals?

| 10% | 20% | 30% | 40% | 50% | 60% | 70% | 80% | 90% | 100% |

MAP IT

FITNESS

	CARDIO	STRENGTH	STRETCHING/ MOBILITY
DAY 1			
DAY 2			
DAY 3			
DAY 4			
DAY 5			
DAY 6			
DAY 7			

NOTES

NUTRITION

	BREAKFAST	LUNCH	DINNER	SNACKS
DAY 1				
DAY 2				
DAY 3				
DAY 4				
DAY 5				
DAY 6				
DAY 7				

NOTES

TRACK IT

DAY 1

Day of the Week/Date _____

TODAY'S FOCUS

☐ Arms ☐ Legs ☐ Core ☐ Chest ☐ Back ☐ Balance ☐ Flexibility ☐ Total-Body Conditioning

CARDIO

ACTIVITY	MINUTES	LEVEL/SPEED/INTENSITY	HEART RATE	CALORIES BURNED	NOTES

STRENGTH

EXERCISE	SET 1		SET 2		SET 3		SET 4		SET 5	
	REPS	WEIGHT	REPS	WEIGHT	REPS	WEIGHT	REPS	WEIGHT	REPS	WEIGHT

STRETCHING/MOBILITY

ACTIVITY/MOVE	REPS/TIME	NOTES

LADDER YOUR REPS. *Laddering helps you tackle reps in a fresh way—especially if you count down. So, for example, start with 5 reps in a set, then 4-3-2-1 with rests in between. Choose the rep-ladder goals that are right for you.*

NUTRITION

	TIME	CALORIES	PROTEIN	CARBS	FAT
BREAKFAST					
SNACK					
LUNCH					
SNACK					
DINNER					
SNACK					
DAILY TOTALS					

WATER (8-OZ SERVINGS)

○ ○ ○ ○ ○ ○ ○ ○ ○ ○ ○ ○ ○ ○ ○

SUPPLEMENT   **AMOUNT**

_____ | _____

_____ | _____

_____ | _____

_____ | _____

_____ | _____

SLEEP

Lights Out _____

Wake Up _____

Quality:

① ② ③ ④ ⑤
⑥ ⑦ ⑧ ⑨ ⑩

RATE YOUR DAY

On track with goals?

| 10% | 20% | 30% | 40% | 50% | 60% | 70% | 80% | 90% | 100% |

TRACK IT

DAY 2

Day of the Week/Date _____

TODAY'S FOCUS

☐ Arms ☐ Legs ☐ Core ☐ Chest ☐ Back ☐ Balance ☐ Flexibility ☐ Total-Body Conditioning

CARDIO

ACTIVITY	MINUTES	LEVEL/SPEED/INTENSITY	HEART RATE	CALORIES BURNED	NOTES

STRENGTH

EXERCISE	SET 1		SET 2		SET 3		SET 4		SET 5	
	REPS	WEIGHT	REPS	WEIGHT	REPS	WEIGHT	REPS	WEIGHT	REPS	WEIGHT

STRETCHING/MOBILITY

ACTIVITY/MOVE	REPS/TIME	NOTES

NOD OFF WITH NUTS. *You'll get your best workout performance when you're well rested. If you have a hard time winding down, try eating more nuts! They're rich in sleep-promoting nutrients such as magnesium and selenium.*

NUTRITION

		TIME	CALORIES	PROTEIN	CARBS	FAT
BREAKFAST						
SNACK						
LUNCH						
SNACK						
DINNER						
SNACK						
DAILY TOTALS						

WATER (8-OZ SERVINGS)

○ ○ ○ ○ ○ ○ ○ ○ ○ ○ ○ ○ ○ ○ ○

SUPPLEMENT	AMOUNT
_____	_____
_____	_____
_____	_____
_____	_____
_____	_____

SLEEP

Lights Out _____

Wake Up _____

Quality:

① ② ③ ④ ⑤
⑥ ⑦ ⑧ ⑨ ⑩

RATE YOUR DAY
On track with goals?

| 10% | 20% | 30% | 40% | 50% | 60% | 70% | 80% | 90% | 100% |

TRACK IT

DAY 3

Day of the Week/Date _____

TODAY'S FOCUS

☐ Arms   ☐ Legs   ☐ Core   ☐ Chest   ☐ Back   ☐ Balance   ☐ Flexibility   ☐ Total-Body Conditioning

CARDIO

ACTIVITY	MINUTES	LEVEL/SPEED/INTENSITY	HEART RATE	CALORIES BURNED	NOTES

STRENGTH

EXERCISE	SET 1		SET 2		SET 3		SET 4		SET 5	
	REPS	WEIGHT	REPS	WEIGHT	REPS	WEIGHT	REPS	WEIGHT	REPS	WEIGHT

STRETCHING/MOBILITY

ACTIVITY/MOVE	REPS/TIME	NOTES

PUSH IT.

"Most people never run far enough on their first wind to find out they've got a second." —William James

NUTRITION

		TIME	CALORIES	PROTEIN	CARBS	FAT
BREAKFAST						
SNACK						
LUNCH						
SNACK						
DINNER						
SNACK						
DAILY TOTALS						

WATER (8-OZ SERVINGS)

○ ○ ○ ○ ○ ○ ○ ○ ○ ○ ○ ○ ○ ○ ○

SUPPLEMENT	AMOUNT
_____	_____
_____	_____
_____	_____
_____	_____
_____	_____

SLEEP

Lights Out _____

Wake Up _____

Quality:

① ② ③ ④ ⑤
⑥ ⑦ ⑧ ⑨ ⑩

RATE YOUR DAY

On track with goals?

10%   20%   30%   40%   50%   60%   70%   80%   90%   100%

DAY 4

Day of the Week/Date _____

TODAY'S FOCUS

☐ Arms ☐ Legs ☐ Core ☐ Chest ☐ Back ☐ Balance ☐ Flexibility ☐ Total-Body Conditioning

CARDIO

ACTIVITY	MINUTES	LEVEL/SPEED/INTENSITY	HEART RATE	CALORIES BURNED	NOTES

STRENGTH

EXERCISE	SET 1		SET 2		SET 3		SET 4		SET 5	
	REPS	WEIGHT	REPS	WEIGHT	REPS	WEIGHT	REPS	WEIGHT	REPS	WEIGHT

STRETCHING/MOBILITY

ACTIVITY/MOVE	REPS/TIME	NOTES

TALK TO YOURSELF. *Motivational self-talk (think: "I've got this!") improved time to exhaustion by 18 percent in a cycling test. Never underestimate the power of mental energy to translate to physical output.*

NUTRITION

		TIME	CALORIES	PROTEIN	CARBS	FAT
BREAKFAST						
SNACK						
LUNCH						
SNACK						
DINNER						
SNACK						
DAILY TOTALS						

WATER (8-OZ SERVINGS)

○ ○ ○ ○ ○ ○ ○ ○ ○ ○ ○ ○ ○ ○ ○ ○

SUPPLEMENT	**AMOUNT**
_____	_____
_____	_____
_____	_____
_____	_____
_____	_____

SLEEP

Lights Out _____

Wake Up _____

Quality:

① ② ③ ④ ⑤
⑥ ⑦ ⑧ ⑨ ⑩

RATE YOUR DAY
On track with goals?

| 10% | 20% | 30% | 40% | 50% | 60% | 70% | 80% | 90% | 100% |

TRACK IT

DAY 5

Day of the Week/Date _____

TODAY'S FOCUS

☐ Arms ☐ Legs ☐ Core ☐ Chest ☐ Back ☐ Balance ☐ Flexibility ☐ Total-Body Conditioning

CARDIO

ACTIVITY	MINUTES	LEVEL/SPEED/INTENSITY	HEART RATE	CALORIES BURNED	NOTES

STRENGTH

EXERCISE	SET 1		SET 2		SET 3		SET 4		SET 5	
	REPS	WEIGHT	REPS	WEIGHT	REPS	WEIGHT	REPS	WEIGHT	REPS	WEIGHT

STRETCHING/MOBILITY

ACTIVITY/MOVE	REPS/TIME	NOTES

GET A GRIP. *Increasing the challenge to your grip recruits more muscles in your hands and forearms. Easiest way to do this: Wrap a towel around the bar or dumbbell handle to make the grip thicker.*

NUTRITION

		TIME	CALORIES	PROTEIN	CARBS	FAT
BREAKFAST						
SNACK						
LUNCH						
SNACK						
DINNER						
SNACK						
DAILY TOTALS						

WATER (8-OZ SERVINGS)

○ ○ ○ ○ ○ ○ ○ ○ ○ ○ ○ ○ ○ ○ ○

SUPPLEMENT   **AMOUNT**

_____ | _____

_____ | _____

_____ | _____

_____ | _____

_____ | _____

SLEEP

Lights Out _____

Wake Up _____

Quality:

① ② ③ ④ ⑤
⑥ ⑦ ⑧ ⑨ ⑩

RATE YOUR DAY

On track with goals?

| 10% 20% 30% 40% 50% 60% 70% 80% 90% 100% |

DAY 6

Day of the Week/Date _____

TODAY'S FOCUS

☐ Arms ☐ Legs ☐ Core ☐ Chest ☐ Back ☐ Balance ☐ Flexibility ☐ Total-Body Conditioning

CARDIO

ACTIVITY	MINUTES	LEVEL/SPEED/INTENSITY	HEART RATE	CALORIES BURNED	NOTES

STRENGTH

EXERCISE	SET 1		SET 2		SET 3		SET 4		SET 5	
	REPS	WEIGHT	REPS	WEIGHT	REPS	WEIGHT	REPS	WEIGHT	REPS	WEIGHT

STRETCHING/MOBILITY

ACTIVITY/MOVE	REPS/TIME	NOTES

MAKE IT HAPPEN.

"Life has no remote. Get up and change it yourself." —Mark A. Cooper

NUTRITION

		TIME	CALORIES	PROTEIN	CARBS	FAT
BREAKFAST						
SNACK						
LUNCH						
SNACK						
DINNER						
SNACK						
	DAILY TOTALS					

WATER (8-OZ SERVINGS)

○ ○ ○ ○ ○ ○ ○ ○ ○ ○ ○ ○ ○ ○ ○

SUPPLEMENT	AMOUNT
_____	_____
_____	_____
_____	_____
_____	_____
_____	_____

SLEEP

Lights Out _____

Wake Up _____

Quality:

① ② ③ ④ ⑤
⑥ ⑦ ⑧ ⑨ ⑩

RATE YOUR DAY
On track with goals?

| 10% | 20% | 30% | 40% | 50% | 60% | 70% | 80% | 90% | 100% |

TRACK IT

DAY 7

Day of the Week/Date _____

TODAY'S FOCUS

☐ Arms ☐ Legs ☐ Core ☐ Chest ☐ Back ☐ Balance ☐ Flexibility ☐ Total-Body Conditioning

CARDIO

ACTIVITY	MINUTES	LEVEL/SPEED/ INTENSITY	HEART RATE	CALORIES BURNED	NOTES

STRENGTH

EXERCISE	SET 1		SET 2		SET 3		SET 4		SET 5	
	REPS	WEIGHT	REPS	WEIGHT	REPS	WEIGHT	REPS	WEIGHT	REPS	WEIGHT

STRETCHING/MOBILITY

ACTIVITY/MOVE	REPS/TIME	NOTES

YOU'RE ALMOST THERE! *Just one more week to finish out this training cycle. Take pride in the progress you've made as you record your gains on pages 10 and 11. Is there a healthy way to reward yourself at the end of week 13?*

NUTRITION

		TIME	CALORIES	PROTEIN	CARBS	FAT
BREAKFAST						
SNACK						
LUNCH						
SNACK						
DINNER						
SNACK						
DAILY TOTALS						

WATER (8-OZ SERVINGS)

○ ○ ○ ○ ○ ○ ○ ○ ○ ○ ○ ○ ○ ○ ○

SUPPLEMENT	**AMOUNT**
_____	_____
_____	_____
_____	_____
_____	_____
_____	_____

SLEEP

Lights Out _____

Wake Up _____

Quality:

① ② ③ ④ ⑤
⑥ ⑦ ⑧ ⑨ ⑩

RATE YOUR DAY
On track with goals?

| 10% | 20% | 30% | 40% | 50% | 60% | 70% | 80% | 90% | 100% |

MAP IT

FITNESS

	CARDIO	STRENGTH	STRETCHING/ MOBILITY
DAY 1			
DAY 2			
DAY 3			
DAY 4			
DAY 5			
DAY 6			
DAY 7			

NOTES

NUTRITION

	BREAKFAST	LUNCH	DINNER	SNACKS
DAY 1				
DAY 2				
DAY 3				
DAY 4				
DAY 5				
DAY 6				
DAY 7				

NOTES

_____
_____
_____
_____

DAY 1

Day of the Week/Date _____

TODAY'S FOCUS

☐ Arms ☐ Legs ☐ Core ☐ Chest ☐ Back ☐ Balance ☐ Flexibility ☐ Total-Body Conditioning

CARDIO

ACTIVITY	MINUTES	LEVEL/SPEED/INTENSITY	HEART RATE	CALORIES BURNED	NOTES

STRENGTH

EXERCISE	SET 1		SET 2		SET 3		SET 4		SET 5	
	REPS	WEIGHT	REPS	WEIGHT	REPS	WEIGHT	REPS	WEIGHT	REPS	WEIGHT

STRETCHING/MOBILITY

ACTIVITY/MOVE	REPS/TIME	NOTES

BENCH-PRESS MORE. *Be sure your feet are directly underneath your hips, then slide them out to the sides of the bench a few inches and keeps your heels down. Squeeze through your glutes as you lift.*

NUTRITION

		TIME	CALORIES	PROTEIN	CARBS	FAT
BREAKFAST						
SNACK						
LUNCH						
SNACK						
DINNER						
SNACK						
DAILY TOTALS						

WATER (8-OZ SERVINGS)

○ ○ ○ ○ ○ ○ ○ ○ ○ ○ ○ ○ ○ ○ ○

SUPPLEMENT   **AMOUNT**

_____ : _____

_____ : _____

_____ : _____

_____ : _____

_____ : _____

SLEEP

Lights Out _____

Wake Up _____

Quality:

① ② ③ ④ ⑤
⑥ ⑦ ⑧ ⑨ ⑩

RATE YOUR DAY
On track with goals?

| 10% | 20% | 30% | 40% | 50% | 60% | 70% | 80% | 90% | 100% |

DAY 2

Day of the Week/Date _____

TODAY'S FOCUS

☐ Arms ☐ Legs ☐ Core ☐ Chest ☐ Back ☐ Balance ☐ Flexibility ☐ Total-Body Conditioning

CARDIO

ACTIVITY	MINUTES	LEVEL/SPEED/ INTENSITY	HEART RATE	CALORIES BURNED	NOTES

STRENGTH

EXERCISE	SET 1		SET 2		SET 3		SET 4		SET 5	
	REPS	WEIGHT	REPS	WEIGHT	REPS	WEIGHT	REPS	WEIGHT	REPS	WEIGHT

STRETCHING/MOBILITY

ACTIVITY/MOVE	REPS/TIME	NOTES

TURN TO TURMERIC. *The Asian spice is an anti-inflammatory that can help relieve postworkout soreness. Sprinkle ¼ to ½ teaspoon on scrambled eggs or rice, with some black pepper to help absorption.*

NUTRITION

		TIME	CALORIES	PROTEIN	CARBS	FAT
BREAKFAST						
SNACK						
LUNCH						
SNACK						
DINNER						
SNACK						
DAILY TOTALS						

WATER (8-OZ SERVINGS)

○ ○ ○ ○ ○ ○ ○ ○ ○ ○ ○ ○ ○ ○ ○

SUPPLEMENT **AMOUNT**

_____ _____

_____ _____

_____ _____

_____ _____

_____ _____

SLEEP

Lights Out _____

Wake Up _____

Quality:

① ② ③ ④ ⑤
⑥ ⑦ ⑧ ⑨ ⑩

RATE YOUR DAY

On track with goals?

| 10% | 20% | 30% | 40% | 50% | 60% | 70% | 80% | 90% | 100% |

DAY 3

Day of the Week/Date _____

TODAY'S FOCUS

☐ Arms ☐ Legs ☐ Core ☐ Chest ☐ Back ☐ Balance ☐ Flexibility ☐ Total-Body Conditioning

CARDIO

ACTIVITY	MINUTES	LEVEL/SPEED/INTENSITY	HEART RATE	CALORIES BURNED	NOTES

STRENGTH

EXERCISE	SET 1		SET 2		SET 3		SET 4		SET 5	
	REPS	WEIGHT	REPS	WEIGHT	REPS	WEIGHT	REPS	WEIGHT	REPS	WEIGHT

STRETCHING/MOBILITY

ACTIVITY/MOVE	REPS/TIME	NOTES

KEEP YOUR DESTINATION IN SIGHT.

"If you aren't going all the way, why go at all?" —Joe Namath

NUTRITION

	TIME	CALORIES	PROTEIN	CARBS	FAT
BREAKFAST					
SNACK					
LUNCH					
SNACK					
DINNER					
SNACK					
DAILY TOTALS					

WATER (8-OZ SERVINGS)

○ ○ ○ ○ ○ ○ ○ ○ ○ ○ ○ ○ ○ ○ ○

SUPPLEMENT	AMOUNT
_____	_____
_____	_____
_____	_____
_____	_____
_____	_____

SLEEP

Lights Out _____

Wake Up _____

Quality:

(1) (2) (3) (4) (5)
(6) (7) (8) (9) (10)

RATE YOUR DAY

On track with goals?

| 10% | 20% | 30% | 40% | 50% | 60% | 70% | 80% | 90% | 100% |

DAY 4

Day of the Week/Date _____

TODAY'S FOCUS

☐ Arms ☐ Legs ☐ Core ☐ Chest ☐ Back ☐ Balance ☐ Flexibility ☐ Total-Body Conditioning

CARDIO

ACTIVITY	MINUTES	LEVEL/SPEED/INTENSITY	HEART RATE	CALORIES BURNED	NOTES

STRENGTH

EXERCISE	SET 1		SET 2		SET 3		SET 4		SET 5	
	REPS	WEIGHT	REPS	WEIGHT	REPS	WEIGHT	REPS	WEIGHT	REPS	WEIGHT

STRETCHING/MOBILITY

ACTIVITY/MOVE	REPS/TIME	NOTES

TEST YOUR 1-REP MAX. *You'll see how far you've come in this training cycle—and get a confidence boost as you move toward setting new goals in your next training cycle. Challenge yourself to always do better.*

NUTRITION

		TIME	CALORIES	PROTEIN	CARBS	FAT
BREAKFAST						
SNACK						
LUNCH						
SNACK						
DINNER						
SNACK						
DAILY TOTALS						

WATER (8-OZ SERVINGS)

○ ○ ○ ○ ○ ○ ○ ○ ○ ○ ○ ○ ○ ○ ○ ○

SUPPLEMENT	AMOUNT
_____	_____
_____	_____
_____	_____
_____	_____
_____	_____

SLEEP

Lights Out _____

Wake Up _____

Quality:

① ② ③ ④ ⑤
⑥ ⑦ ⑧ ⑨ ⑩

RATE YOUR DAY
On track with goals?

| 10% | 20% | 30% | 40% | 50% | 60% | 70% | 80% | 90% | 100% |

DAY 5

Day of the Week/Date _____

TODAY'S FOCUS

☐ Arms ☐ Legs ☐ Core ☐ Chest ☐ Back ☐ Balance ☐ Flexibility ☐ Total-Body Conditioning

CARDIO

ACTIVITY	MINUTES	LEVEL/SPEED/INTENSITY	HEART RATE	CALORIES BURNED	NOTES

STRENGTH

EXERCISE	SET 1		SET 2		SET 3		SET 4		SET 5	
	REPS	WEIGHT	REPS	WEIGHT	REPS	WEIGHT	REPS	WEIGHT	REPS	WEIGHT

STRETCHING/MOBILITY

ACTIVITY/MOVE	REPS/TIME	NOTES

GO RED FOR RESULTS. *Pomegranates may give your workout a boost. A study found that 8 ounces of 100 percent pomegranate juice daily increased post-exercise arm and leg strength.*

NUTRITION

	TIME	CALORIES	PROTEIN	CARBS	FAT
BREAKFAST					
SNACK					
LUNCH					
SNACK					
DINNER					
SNACK					
DAILY TOTALS					

WATER (8-OZ SERVINGS)
○ ○ ○ ○ ○ ○ ○ ○ ○ ○ ○ ○ ○ ○ ○

SUPPLEMENT	AMOUNT
_____	_____
_____	_____
_____	_____
_____	_____
_____	_____

SLEEP
Lights Out _____

Wake Up _____

Quality:

① ② ③ ④ ⑤
⑥ ⑦ ⑧ ⑨ ⑩

RATE YOUR DAY
On track with goals?

10%   20%   30%   40%   50%   60%   70%   80%   90%   100%

TRACK IT

DAY 6

Day of the Week/Date _____

TODAY'S FOCUS

☐ Arms ☐ Legs ☐ Core ☐ Chest ☐ Back ☐ Balance ☐ Flexibility ☐ Total-Body Conditioning

CARDIO

ACTIVITY	MINUTES	LEVEL/SPEED/INTENSITY	HEART RATE	CALORIES BURNED	NOTES

STRENGTH

EXERCISE	SET 1		SET 2		SET 3		SET 4		SET 5	
	REPS	WEIGHT	REPS	WEIGHT	REPS	WEIGHT	REPS	WEIGHT	REPS	WEIGHT

STRETCHING/MOBILITY

ACTIVITY/MOVE	REPS/TIME	NOTES

YOU WON'T REGRET YOUR BEST. *"You find that you have peace of mind and can enjoy yourself, get more sleep, and rest when you know that it was a 100 percent effort that you gave—win or lose."* —*Gordie Howe*

NUTRITION

		TIME	CALORIES	PROTEIN	CARBS	FAT
BREAKFAST						
SNACK						
LUNCH						
SNACK						
DINNER						
SNACK						
	DAILY TOTALS					

WATER (8-OZ SERVINGS)

○ ○ ○ ○ ○ ○ ○ ○ ○ ○ ○ ○ ○ ○ ○

SUPPLEMENT   **AMOUNT**

_____

_____

_____

_____

_____

SLEEP

Lights Out _____

Wake Up _____

Quality:

① ② ③ ④ ⑤
⑥ ⑦ ⑧ ⑨ ⑩

RATE YOUR DAY
On track with goals?

| 10% | 20% | 30% | 40% | 50% | 60% | 70% | 80% | 90% | 100% |

TRACK IT

DAY 7

Day of the Week/Date _____

TODAY'S FOCUS

☐ Arms   ☐ Legs   ☐ Core   ☐ Chest   ☐ Back   ☐ Balance   ☐ Flexibility   ☐ Total-Body Conditioning

CARDIO

ACTIVITY	MINUTES	LEVEL/SPEED/INTENSITY	HEART RATE	CALORIES BURNED	NOTES

STRENGTH

EXERCISE	SET 1		SET 2		SET 3		SET 4		SET 5	
	REPS	WEIGHT	REPS	WEIGHT	REPS	WEIGHT	REPS	WEIGHT	REPS	WEIGHT

STRETCHING/MOBILITY

ACTIVITY/MOVE	REPS/TIME	NOTES

FINAL CHECK-IN! *Reward yourself for your hard work! Allow yourself a few days or up to a week of rest, then come back strong into a new training cycle with a new set of goals entered in a fresh workout journal for the journey.*

NUTRITION

		TIME	CALORIES	PROTEIN	CARBS	FAT
BREAKFAST						
SNACK						
LUNCH						
SNACK						
DINNER						
SNACK						
DAILY TOTALS						

WATER (8-OZ SERVINGS)
○ ○ ○ ○ ○ ○ ○ ○ ○ ○ ○ ○ ○ ○ ○ ○

SUPPLEMENT   **AMOUNT**

_____ | _____
_____ | _____
_____ | _____
_____ | _____
_____ | _____

SLEEP

Lights Out _____

Wake Up _____

Quality:

① ② ③ ④ ⑤
⑥ ⑦ ⑧ ⑨ ⑩

RATE YOUR DAY
On track with goals?

| 10% | 20% | 30% | 40% | 50% | 60% | 70% | 80% | 90% | 100% |

"TO ACHIEVE ANYTHING REQUIRES FAITH AND BELIEF IN YOURSELF, VISION, HARD WORK, DETERMINATION, AND DEDICATION. REMEMBER ALL THINGS ARE POSSIBLE FOR THOSE WHO BELIEVE."

—GAIL DEVERS